The Cardiovascular System at a Glance

This new edition is also available as an e-book.
For more details, please see www.wiley.com/buy/9780470655948 or scan this QR code:

Companion website

A companion website is available at:

www.ataglanceseries.com/cardiovascular

featuring:
- Case Studies from this and previous editions
- Key points for revision

The Cardiovascular System at a Glance

Philip I. Aaronson

BA, PhD
Reader in Pharmacology and Therapeutics
Division of Asthma, Allergy and Lung Biology
King's College London
London

Jeremy P.T. Ward

BSc, PhD
Head of Department of Physiology and Professor of Respiratory Cell Physiology
King's College London
London

Michelle J. Connolly

BSc, MBBS, AKC, PhD
Academic Foundation Doctor
Royal Free Hospital
London

Fourth Edition

WILEY-BLACKWELL

A John Wiley & Sons, Ltd., Publication

This edition first published 2013 © 2013 by John Wiley & Sons, Ltd
Previous editions 1999, 2004, 2007

Blackwell Publishing was acquired by John Wiley & Sons in February 2007. Blackwell's publishing program has been merged with Wiley's global Scientific, Technical and Medical business to form Wiley-Blackwell.

Registered office: John Wiley & Sons, Ltd, The Atrium, Southern Gate, Chichester, West Sussex, PO19 8SQ, UK

Editorial offices: 9600 Garsington Road, Oxford, OX4 2DQ, UK
The Atrium, Southern Gate, Chichester, West Sussex, PO19 8SQ, UK
350 Main Street, Malden, MA 02148-5020, USA

For details of our global editorial offices, for customer services and for information about how to apply for permission to reuse the copyright material in this book please see our website at www.wiley.com/wiley-blackwell.

The right of the authors to be identified as the authors of this work has been asserted in accordance with the UK Copyright, Designs and Patents Act 1988.

Library of Congress Cataloging-in-Publication Data
Aaronson, Philip I. (Philip Irving), 1953–
  The cardiovascular system at a glance / Philip I. Aaronson, Jeremy P.T. Ward,
Michelle J. Connolly. – 4th ed.
      p. cm.
  Includes bibliographical references and index.
  ISBN 978-0-470-65594-8 (pbk. : alk. paper)   1. Cardiovascular system–Physiology.
2. Cardiovascular system–Pathophysiology.   I. Ward, Jeremy P. T.   II. Connolly, Michelle J.
III. Title.
  QP101.C293 2013
  612.1–dc23

                           2012024674

A catalogue record for this book is available from the British Library.
Cover image: Getty images
Cover design by Meaden Creative

Wiley also publishes its books in a variety of electronic formats. Some content that appears in print may not be available in electronic books.

Set in 9/11.5 pt Times by Toppan Best-set Premedia Limited
Printed and bound in Malaysia by Vivar Printing Sdn Bhd

3   2016

Contents

A companion website is available for this book at: www.ataglanceseries.com/cardiovascular

Preface

This book is designed to present a concise description of the cardiovascular system which integrates normal structure and function with pathophysiology, pharmacology and therapeutics. We therefore cover in an accessible yet comprehensive manner all of the topics that preclinical medical students and biomedical science students are likely to encounter when they are learning about the cardiovascular system. However, our aims in writing and revising this book have always been more ambitious – we have also sought to provide to our readers a straightforward description of many fascinating and important topics that are neglected or covered only superficially by many other textbooks and most university and medical courses. We hope that this book will not only inform you about the cardiovascular system, but enthuse you to look more deeply into at least some of its many remarkable aspects.

In addition to making substantial revisions designed to update the topics, address reviewers' criticisms and simplify some of the diagrams, we have added a new chapter on pulmonary hypertension for this fourth edition and written eight entirely new self-assessment case studies, each drawing on encounters with real patients.

Philip I. Aaronson
Jeremy P.T. Ward
Michelle J. Connolly

Recommended reading

Bonow R.O., Mann D.L., Zipes D.P. & Libby P. (Eds) (2011) *Braunwald's Heart Disease: A Textbook of Cardiovascular Medicine*, 9th edition. Elsevier Health Sciences.

Levick J.R. (2010) *An Introduction to Cardiovascular Physiology*, 5th edition. Hodder Arnold.

Lilly L.S. (Ed). (2010) *Pathophysiology of Heart Disease: A Collaborative Project of Medical Students and Faculty*, 5th edition. Lippincott Williams and Wilkins.

Acknowledgements

We are most grateful to Dr Daniela Sergi, consultant in acute medicine at North Middlesex University Hospital NHS Trust, and Dr Paul E. Pfeffer, specialist registrar and clinical research fellow at Guy's and St Thomas' NHS Foundation Trust for reviewing the clinical chapters and case studies.

We would also like to thank Professor Horst Olschewski and Dr Gabor Kovacs, internationally renowned experts on pulmonary hypertension at the Ludwig Boltzmann Institute for Lung Vascular Research at the Medical University of Graz, Austria, for writing the new case study on pulmonary arterial hypertension.

We are grateful to Karen Moore for her assistance in keeping track of our progress, putting up so gracefully with our missed deadlines, and generally making sure that this book and its companion website not only became a reality, but did so on schedule. Finally, as always, we thank our readers, particularly our students at King's College London, whose support over the years has encouraged us to keep trying to make this book better.

List of abbreviations

5-HT	5-hydroxytryptamine (serotonin)
AAA	abdominal aortic aneurysm
ABP	arterial blood pressure
AC	adenylate cyclase
ACE	angiotensin-converting enzyme
ACEI	angiotensin-converting enzyme inhibitor/s
ACS	acute coronary syndromes
ADH	antidiuretic hormone
ADMA	asymmetrical dimethyl arginine
ADP	adenosine diphosphate
AF	atrial fibrillation
AMP	adenosine monophosphate
ANP	atrial natriuretic peptide
ANS	autonomic nervous system
AP	action potential
APAH	pulmonary hypertension associated with other conditions
APC	active protein C
APD	action potential duration
aPTT	activated partial thromboplastin time
AR	aortic regurgitation
ARB	angiotensin II receptor blocker
ARDS	acute respiratory distress syndrome
AS	aortic stenosis
ASD	atrial septal defect
ATP	adenosine triphosphate
AV	atrioventricular
AVA	arteriovenous anastomosis
AVN	atrioventricular node
AVNRT	atrioventricular nodal re-entrant tachycardia
AVRT	atrioventricular re-entrant tachycardia
BBB	blood–brain barrier
BP	blood pressure
CABG	coronary artery bypass grafting
CAD	coronary artery disease
CaM	calmodulin
cAMP	cyclic adenosine monophosphate
CCB	calcium-channel blocker
CE	cholesteryl ester
CETP	cholesteryl ester transfer protein
CFU-E	colony-forming unit erythroid cell
cGMP	cyclic guanosine monophosphate
CHD	congenital heart disease
CHD	coronary heart disease
CHF	chronic heart failure
CICR	calcium-induced calcium release
CK-MB	creatine kinase MB
CNS	central nervous system
CO	cardiac output
COPD	chronic obstructive pulmonary disease
COX	cyclooxygenase
CPVT	catecholaminergic polymorphic ventricular tachycardia
CRP	C-reactive protein
CSF	cerebrospinal fluid
CT	computed tomography
CTPA	computed tomography pulmonary angiogram
CVD	cardiovascular disease
CVP	central venous pressure
CXR	chest X-ray
DAD	delayed afterdepolarization
DAG	diacylglycerol
DBP	diastolic blood pressure
DC	direct current
DHP	dihydropyridine
DIC	disseminated intravascular coagulation
DM2	type 2 diabetes mellitus
DVT	deep venous/vein thrombosis
EAD	early afterdepolarization
ECF	extracellular fluid
ECG	electrocardiogram/electrocardiograph (EKG)
ECM	extracellular matrix
EDHF	endothelium-derived hyperpolarizing factor
EDP	end-diastolic pressure
EDRF	endothelium-derived relaxing factor
EDTA	ethylenediaminetetraacetic acid
EDV	end-diastolic volume
EET	epoxyeicosatrienoic acid
EnaC	epithelial sodium channel
eNOS	endothelial NOS
ERP	effective refractory period
ESR	erythrocyte sedimentation rate
FDP	fibrin degradation product
GP	glycoprotein
GPI	glycoprotein inhibitor
GTN	glyceryl trinitrate
Hb	haemoglobin
HCM	hypertrophic cardiomyopathy
HDL	high-density lipoprotein
HEET	hydroxyeicosatetraenoic acid
HMG-CoA	hydroxy-methylglutanyl coenzyme A
hPAH	heritable pulmonary arterial hypertension
HPV	hypoxic pulmonary vasoconstriction
HR	heart rate
ICD	implantable cardioverter defibrillator
IDL	intermediate-density lipoprotein
Ig	immunoglobulin
IML	intermediolateral
iNOS	inducible NOS
INR	international normalized ratio
IP$_3$	inisotol 1,4,5-triphosphate
iPAH	idiopathic pulmonary arterial hypertension
ISH	isolated systolic hypertension
JVP	jugular venous pressure
LA	left atrium
LDL	low-density lipoprotein
LITA	left internal thoracic artery
LMWH	low molecular weight heparin
L-NAME	L-nitro arginine methyl ester
LPL	lipoprotein lipase

LQT	long QT
LV	left ventricle/left ventricular
LVH	left ventricular hypertrophy
MABP	mean arterial blood pressure
MCH	mean cell haemoglobin
MCHC	mean cell haemoglobin concentration
MCV	mean cell volume
MI	myocardial infarction
MLCK	myosin light-chain kinase
mPAP	mean pressure in the pulmonary artery
MR	mitral regurgitation
MRI	magnetic resonance imaging
MS	mitral stenosis
MW	molecular weight
NCX	Na^+–Ca^{2+} exchanger
NK	natural killer
NO	nitric oxide
NOS	nitric oxide synthase
nNOS	neuronal nitric oxide synthase
NSAID	non-steroidal anti-inflammatory drug
NSCC	non-selective cation channel
NSTEMI	non-ST segment elevation myocardial infarction
NTS	nucleus tractus solitarius
NYHA	New York Heart Association
PA	postero-anterior
PA	pulmonary artery
PAH	pulmonary arterial hypertension
PAI-1	plasminogen activator inhibitor-1
PCI	percutaneous coronary intervention
PCV	packed cell volume
PD	potential difference
PDA	patent ductus arteriosus
PDE	phosphodiesterase
PE	pulmonary embolism
PGE$_2$	prostaglandin E_2
PGI$_2$	prostacyclin
PH	pulmonary hypertension
PI3K	phosphatidylinositol 3-kinase
PKA	protein kinase A
PKC	protein kinase C
PKG	cyclic GMP-dependent protein kinase
PLD	phospholipid
PMCA	plasma membrane Ca^{2+}-ATPase
PMN	polymorphonuclear leucocyte
PND	paroxysmal nocturnal dyspnoea
PPAR	proliferator-activated receptor
PRU	peripheral resistance unit
PT	prothrombin time
PTCA	percutaneous transcoronary angioplasty
PVC	premature ventricular contraction
PVR	pulmonary vascular resistance
RAA	renin–angiotensin–aldosterone
RCA	radiofrequency catheter ablation
RCC	red cell count
RGC	receptor-gated channel
RMP	resting membrane potential
RV	right ventricle/right ventricular
RVLM	rostral ventrolateral medulla
RVOT	right ventricular outflow tract tachycardia
RyR	ryanodine receptor
SAN	sinoatrial node
SERCA	smooth endoplasmic reticulum Ca^{2+}-ATPase
SHO	senior house officer
SK	streptokinase
SMTC	S-methyl-L-thiocitrulline
SOC	store-operated Ca^{2+} channel
SPECT	single photon emission computed tomography
SR	sarcoplasmic reticulum
STEMI	ST elevation myocardial infarction
SV	stroke volume
SVR	systemic vascular resistance
SVT	supraventricular tachycardia
TAFI	thrombin activated fibrinolysis inhibitor
TAVI	transcatheter aortic valve implantation
TB	tuberculosis
TEE	transthoracic echocardiogram
TF	tissue factor thromboplastin
TFPI	tissue factor pathway inhibitor
TGF	transforming growth factor
TOE	transoesophageal echocardiography/echocardiogram
tPA	tissue plasminogen activator
TPR	total peripheral resistance
TRP	transient receptor potential
TXA$_2$	thromboxane A_2
UA	unstable angina
uPA	urokinase
VF	ventricular fibrillation
VGC	voltage-gated channel
VLDL	very low density lipoprotein
VSD	ventricular septal defect
VSM	vascular smooth muscle
VT	ventricular tachycardia
VTE	venous thromboembolism
vWF	von Willebrand factor
WBCC	white blood cell count
WPW	Wolff–Parkinson–White

1 Overview of the cardiovascular system

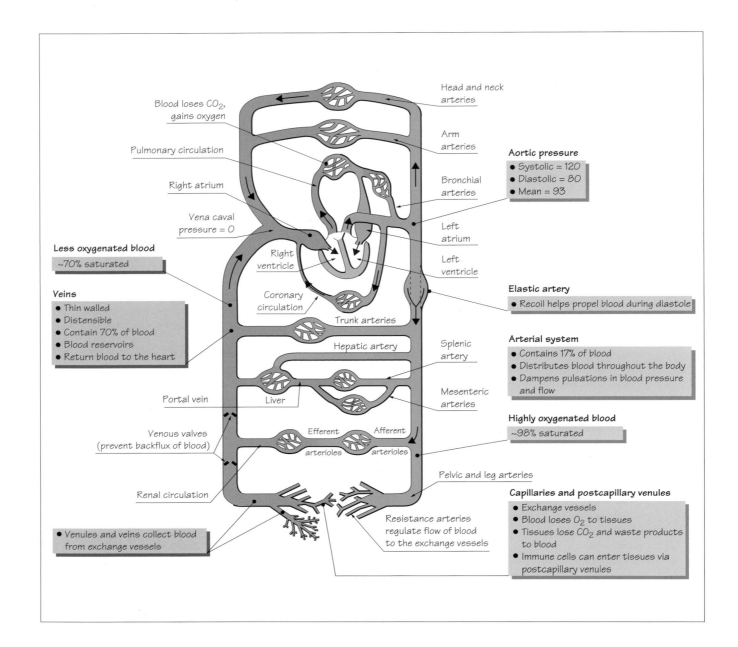

The cardiovascular system is composed of the heart, blood vessels and blood. In simple terms, its main functions are:

1 distribution of O_2 and nutrients (e.g. glucose, amino acids) to all body tissues

2 transportation of CO_2 and metabolic waste products (e.g. urea) from the tissues to the lungs and excretory organs

3 distribution of water, electrolytes and hormones throughout the body

4 contributing to the infrastructure of the immune system

5 thermoregulation.

Blood is composed of **plasma**, an aqueous solution containing electrolytes, proteins and other molecules, in which **cells** are suspended. The cells comprise 40–45% of blood volume and are mainly **erythrocytes**, but also **white blood cells** and **platelets**. Blood volume is about 5.5 L in an 'average' 70-kg man.

Figure 1 illustrates the 'plumbing' of the cardiovascular system.

Blood is driven through the cardiovascular system by the **heart**, a muscular pump divided into left and right sides. Each side contains two chambers, an **atrium** and a **ventricle**, composed mainly of cardiac muscle cells. The thin-walled atria serve to fill or 'prime'

The Cardiovascular System at a Glance, Fourth Edition. Philip I. Aaronson, Jeremy P.T. Ward, and Michelle J. Connolly.

the thick-walled ventricles, which when full constrict forcefully, creating a pressure head that drives the blood out into the body. Blood enters and leaves each chamber of the heart through separate one-way valves, which open and close reciprocally (i.e. one closes before the other opens) to ensure that flow is unidirectional.

Consider the flow of blood, starting with its exit from the left ventricle.

When the ventricles contract, the left ventricular internal pressure rises from 0 to 120 mmHg (atmospheric pressure = 0). As the pressure rises, the aortic valve opens and blood is expelled into the **aorta**, the first and largest artery of the **systemic circulation**. This period of ventricular contraction is termed **systole**. The maximal pressure during systole is called the **systolic pressure**, and it serves both to drive blood through the aorta and to distend the aorta, which is quite elastic. The aortic valve then closes, and the left ventricle relaxes so that it can be refilled with blood from the left atrium via the mitral valve. The period of relaxation is called **diastole**. During diastole aortic blood flow and pressure diminish but do not fall to zero, because *elastic recoil* of the aorta continues to exert a **diastolic pressure** on the blood, which gradually falls to a minimum level of about 80 mmHg. The difference between systolic and diastolic pressures is termed the **pulse pressure**. **Mean arterial blood pressure** (MABP) is pressure averaged over the entire cardiac cycle. Because the heart spends approximately 60% of the cardiac cycle in diastole, the MABP is approximately equal to the diastolic pressure + one-third of the pulse pressure, rather than to the arithmetic average of the systolic and diastolic pressures.

The blood flows from the aorta into the **major arteries**, each of which supplies blood to an organ or body region. These arteries divide and subdivide into smaller **muscular arteries**, which eventually give rise to the **arterioles** – arteries with diameters of <100 μm. Blood enters the arterioles at a mean pressure of about 60–70 mmHg.

The walls of the arteries and arterioles have circumferentially arranged layers of **smooth muscle cells**. The lumen of the entire vascular system is lined by a monolayer of **endothelial cells**. These cells secrete vasoactive substances and serve as a barrier, restricting and controlling the movement of fluid, molecules and cells into and out of the vasculature.

The arterioles lead to the smallest vessels, the **capillaries**, which form a dense network within all body tissues. The capillary wall is a layer of overlapping endothelial cells, with no smooth muscle cells. The pressure in the capillaries ranges from about 25 mmHg on the arterial side to 15 mmHg at the venous end. The capillaries converge into small **venules**, which also have thin walls of mainly endothelial cells. The venules merge into larger venules, with an increasing content of smooth muscle cells as they widen. These then converge to become **veins**, which progressively join to give rise to the **superior** and **inferior venae cavae**, through which blood returns to the right side of the heart. Veins have a larger diameter than arteries, and thus offer relatively little resistance to flow. The

small pressure gradient between venules (15 mmHg) and the venae cavae (0 mmHg) is therefore sufficient to drive blood back to the heart.

Blood from the venae cavae enters the **right atrium**, and then the **right ventricle** through the **tricuspid valve**. Contraction of the right ventricle, simultaneous with that of the left ventricle, forces blood through the pulmonary valve into the pulmonary artery, which progressively subdivides to form the arteries, arterioles and capillaries of the **pulmonary circulation**. The pulmonary circulation is shorter and has a much lower pressure than the systemic circulation, with systolic and diastolic pressures of about 25 and 10 mmHg, respectively. The pulmonary capillary network within the lungs surrounds the alveoli of the lungs, allowing exchange of CO_2 for O_2. Oxygenated blood enters pulmonary venules and veins, and then the **left atrium**, which pumps it into the left ventricle for the next systemic cycle.

The output of the right ventricle is slightly lower than that of the left ventricle. This is because 1–2% of the systemic blood flow never reaches the right atrium, but is shunted to the left side of the heart via the bronchial circulation (Figure 1) and a small fraction of coronary blood flow drains into the thebesian veins (see Chapter 2).

Blood vessel functions

Each vessel type has important functions in addition to being a conduit for blood.

The branching system of elastic and muscular arteries progressively reduces the pulsations in blood pressure and flow imposed by the intermittent ventricular contractions.

The smallest arteries and arterioles have a crucial role in regulating the amount of blood flowing to the tissues by dilating or constricting. This function is regulated by the sympathetic nervous system, and factors generated locally in tissues. These vessels are referred to as **resistance arteries**, because their constriction resists the flow of blood.

Capillaries and small venules are the **exchange vessels**. Through their walls, gases, fluids and molecules are transferred between blood and tissues. White blood cells can also pass through the venule walls to fight infection in the tissues.

Venules can constrict to offer resistance to the blood flow, and the ratio of arteriolar and venular resistance exerts an important influence on the movement of fluid between capillaries and tissues, thereby affecting blood volume.

The veins are thin walled and very *distensible*, and therefore contain about 70% of all blood in the cardiovascular system. The arteries contain just 17% of total blood volume. Veins and venules thus serve as volume reservoirs, which can shift blood from the peripheral circulation into the heart and arteries by constricting. In doing so, they can help to increase the **cardiac output** (volume of blood pumped by the heart per unit time), and they are also able to maintain the blood pressure and tissue perfusion in essential organs if **haemorrhage** (blood loss) occurs.

Gross anatomy and histology of the heart

2

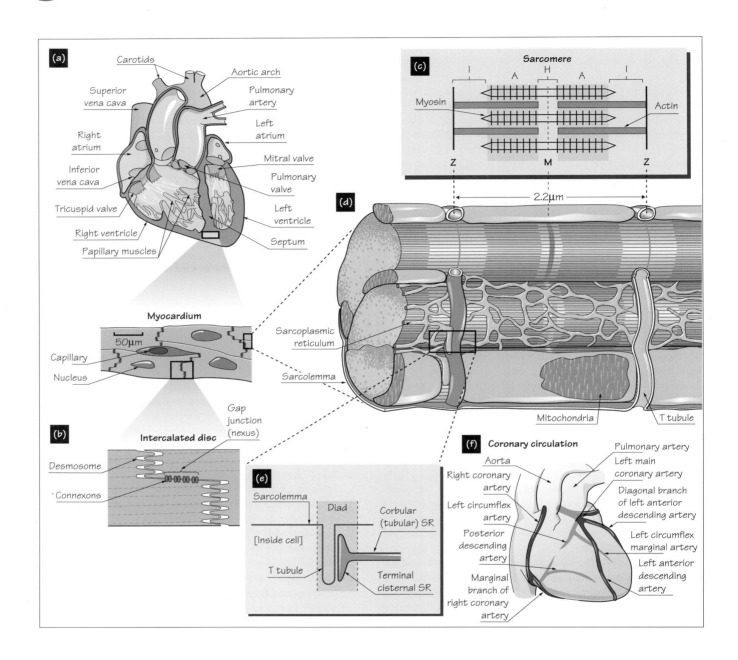

The Cardiovascular System at a Glance, Fourth Edition. Philip I. Aaronson, Jeremy P.T. Ward, and Michelle J. Connolly.
© 2013 John Wiley & Sons, Ltd. Published 2013 by John Wiley & Sons, Ltd.

Gross anatomy of the heart (Figure 2a)

The heart consists of four chambers. Blood flows into the right atrium via the superior and inferior venae cavae. The left and right atria connect to the ventricles via the mitral (two cusps) and tricuspid (three cusps) atrioventricular (AV) valves, respectively. The AV valves are passive and close when the ventricular pressure exceeds that in the atrium. They are prevented from being everted into the atria during systole by fine cords (**chordae tendineae**) attached between the free margins of the cusps and the papillary muscles, which contract during systole. The outflow from the right ventricle passes through the pulmonary semilunar valve to the pulmonary artery, and that from the left ventricle enters the aorta via the aortic semilunar valve. These valves close passively at the end of systole, when ventricular pressure falls below that of the arteries. Both semilunar valves have three cusps.

The cusps or leaflets of the cardiac valves are formed of fibrous connective tissue, covered in a thin layer of cells similar to and contiguous with the **endocardium** (AV valves and ventricular surface of semilunar valves) and **endothelium** (vascular side of semilunar valves). When closed, the cusps form a tight seal (come to apposition) at the **commissures** (line at which the edges of the leaflets meet).

The atria and ventricles are separated by a band of fibrous connective tissue called the **annulus fibrosus**, which provides a skeleton for attachment of the muscle and insertion of the valves. It also prevents electrical conduction between the atria and ventricles except at the **atrioventricular node** (AVN). This is situated near the interatrial septum and the mouth of the coronary sinus and is an important element of the cardiac electrical conduction system (see Chapter 13).

The ventricles fill during diastole; at the initiation of the heart beat the atria contract and complete ventricular filling. As the ventricles contract the pressure rises sharply, closing the AV valves. When ventricular pressure exceeds the pulmonary artery or aortic pressure, the semilunar valves open and ejection occurs (see Chapter 16). As systole ends and ventricular pressure falls, the semilunar valves are closed by backflow of blood from the arteries.

The force of contraction is generated by the muscle of the heart, the **myocardium**. The atrial walls are thin. The greater pressure generated by the left ventricle compared with the right is reflected by its greater wall thickness. The inside of the heart is covered in a thin layer of cells called the **endocardium**, which is similar to the endothelium of blood vessels. The outer surface of the myocardium is covered by the **epicardium**, a layer of mesothelial cells. The whole heart is enclosed in the **pericardium**, a thin fibrous sheath or sac, which prevents excessive enlargement. The **pericardial space** contains interstitial fluid as a lubricant.

Structure of the myocardium

The myocardium consists of **cardiac myocytes** (*muscle cells*) that show a striated subcellular structure, although they are less organized than skeletal muscle. The cells are relatively small ($100 \times 20\,\mu m$) and branched, with a single nucleus, and are rich in mitochondria. They are connected together as a network by **intercalated discs** (Figure 2b), where the cell membranes are closely opposed. The intercalated discs provide both a structural attachment by 'glueing' the cells together at **desmosomes**, and an electrical connection through **gap junctions** formed of pores made up of proteins called **connexons**. As a result, the myocardium acts as a **functional syncytium**, in other words as a single functional unit, even though the individual cells are still separate. The gap junctions play a vital part in conduction of the electrical impulse through the myocardium (see Chapter 13).

The myocytes contain **actin** and **myosin** filaments which form the contractile apparatus, and exhibit the classic M and Z lines and A, H and I bands (Figure 2c). The intercalated discs always coincide with a Z line, as it is here that the actin filaments are anchored to the cytoskeleton. At the Z lines the **sarcolemma** (cell membrane) forms tubular invaginations into the cells known as the **transverse (T) tubular system**. The **sarcoplasmic reticulum** (SR) is less extensive than in skeletal muscle, and runs generally in parallel with the length of the cell (Figure 2d). Close to the T tubules the SR forms **terminal cisternae** that with the T tubule make up **diads** (Figure 2e), an important component of excitation–contraction coupling (see Chapter 12). The typical *triad* seen in skeletal muscle is less often present. The T tubules and SR never physically join, but are separated by a narrow gap. The myocardium has an extensive system of capillaries.

Coronary circulation (Figure 2f)

The heart has a rich blood supply, derived from the **left and right coronary arteries**. These arise separately from the aortic sinus at the base of the aorta, behind the cusps of the aortic valve. They are not blocked by the cusps during systole because of eddy currents, and remain patent throughout the cardiac cycle. The **right coronary artery** runs forward between the pulmonary trunk and right atrium, to the AV sulcus. As it descends to the lower margin of the heart, it divides to **posterior descending** and **right marginal** branches. The **left coronary artery** runs behind the pulmonary trunk and forward between it and the left atrium. It divides into the **circumflex**, **left marginal** and **anterior descending** branches. There are anastomoses between the left and right marginal branches, and the anterior and posterior descending arteries, although these are not sufficient to maintain perfusion if one side of the coronary circulation is occluded.

Most of the blood returns to the right atrium via the **coronary sinus**, and **anterior cardiac veins**. The **large** and **small** coronary veins run parallel to the left and right coronary arteries, respectively, and empty into the sinus. Numerous other small vessels empty into the cardiac chambers directly, including **thebesian veins** and **arteriosinusoidal vessels**.

The coronary circulation is capable of developing a good collateral system in ischaemic heart disease, when a branch or branches are occluded by, for example, atheromatous plaques. Most of the left ventricle is supplied by the left coronary artery, and occlusion can therefore be very dangerous. The AVN and **sinus node** are supplied by the right coronary artery in the majority of people; disease in this artery can cause a slow heart rate and AV block (see Chapters 13 and 14).

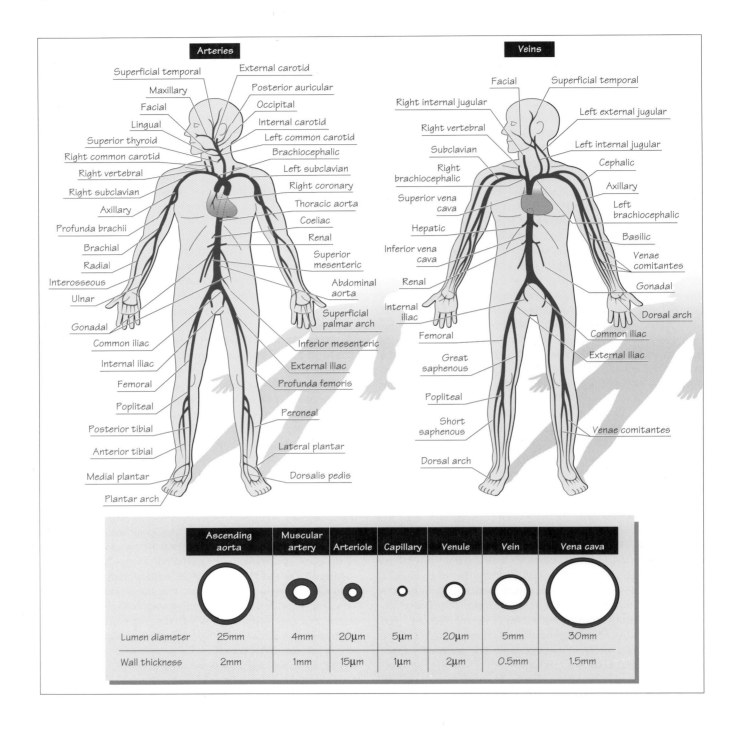

	Ascending aorta	Muscular artery	Arteriole	Capillary	Venule	Vein	Vena cava
Lumen diameter	25mm	4mm	20μm	5μm	20μm	5mm	30mm
Wall thickness	2mm	1mm	15μm	1μm	2μm	0.5mm	1.5mm

The Cardiovascular System at a Glance, Fourth Edition. Philip I. Aaronson, Jeremy P.T. Ward, and Michelle J. Connolly.

The blood vessels of the cardiovascular system are for convenience of description classified into **arteries** (elastic and muscular), **resistance vessels** (small arteries and arterioles), **capillaries**, **venules** and **veins**. Typical dimensions for the different types of vessel are illustrated.

The systemic circulation
Arteries
The **systemic (or greater) circulation** begins with the pumping of blood by the left ventricle into the largest artery, the **aorta**. This ascends from the top of the heart, bends downward at the **aortic arch** and descends just anterior to the spinal column. The aorta bifurcates into the left and right **iliac arteries**, which supply the pelvis and legs. The major arteries supplying the head, the arms and the heart arise from the aortic arch, and the main arteries supplying the visceral organs branch from the descending aorta. All of the major organs except the liver (see below) are therefore supplied with blood by arteries that arise from the aorta. The fundamentally *parallel* organization of the systemic vasculature has a number of advantages over the alternative *series* arrangement, in which blood would flow sequentially through one organ after another. The parallel arrangement of the vascular system ensures that the supply of blood to each organ is relatively independent, is driven by a large pressure head, and also that each organ receives highly oxygenated blood.

The aorta and its major branches (**brachiocephalic**, **common carotid**, **subclavian** and **common iliac** arteries) are termed **elastic arteries**. In addition to conducting blood away from the heart, these arteries distend during systole and recoil during diastole, damping the pulse wave and evening out the discontinuous flow of blood created by the heart's intermittent pumping action.

Elastic arteries branch to give rise to **muscular arteries** with relatively thicker walls; this prevents their collapse when joints bend. The muscular arteries give rise to **resistance vessels**, so named because they present the greatest part of the resistance of the vasculature to the flow of blood. These are sometimes subclassified into small arteries, which have multiple layers of smooth muscle cells in their walls, and **arterioles**, which have one or two layers of smooth muscle cells. Resistance vessels have the highest wall to lumen ratio in the vasculature. The degree of constriction or tone of these vessels regulates the amount of blood flowing to each small area of tissue. All but the smallest resistance vessels tend to be heavily innervated (especially in the *splanchnic*, *renal* and *cutaneous* vasculatures) by the **sympathetic nervous system**, the activity of which usually causes them to constrict (see Chapter 28).

Arterial anastomoses
In addition to branching to give rise to smaller vessels, arteries and arterioles may also merge to form **anastomoses**. These are found in many circulations (e.g. the brain, mesentery, uterus, around joints) and provide an alternative supply of blood if one artery is blocked. If this occurs, the anastamosing artery gradually enlarges, providing a **collateral circulation**.

The smallest arterioles, capillaries and postcapillary venules comprise the **microcirculation**, the structure and function of which is described in Chapters 20 and 21.

Veins
The venous system can be divided into the **venules**, which contain one or two layers of smooth muscle cells, and the **veins**. The veins of the limbs, particularly the legs, contain paired **semilunar valves** which ensure that the blood cannot move backwards. These are orientated so that they are pressed against the venous wall when the blood is flowing forward, but are forced out to occlude the lumen when the blood flow reverses.

The veins from the head, neck and arms come together to form the **superior vena cava**, and those from the lower part of the body merge into the **inferior vena cava**. These deliver blood to the right atrium, which pumps it into the right ventricle.

The one or two veins draining a body region typically run next to the artery supplying that region. This promotes heat conservation, because at low temperatures the warmer arterial blood gives up its heat to the cooler venous blood, rather than to the external environment. The pulsations of the artery caused by the heart beat also aid the venous flow of blood.

The pulmonary circulation
The **pulmonary (or lesser) circulation** begins when blood is pumped by the right ventricle into the **main pulmonary artery**, which immediately bifurcates into the **right** and **left pulmonary arteries** supplying each lung. This 'venous' blood is oxygenated during its passage through the pulmonary capillaries. It then returns to the heart via the **pulmonary veins** to the left atrium, which pumps it into the left ventricle. The metabolic demands of the lungs are not met by the pulmonary circulation, but by the **bronchial circulation**. This arises from the **intercostal arteries**, which branch from the aorta. Most of the veins of the bronchial circulation terminate in the right atrium, but some drain into the pulmonary veins (see Chapter 26).

The splanchnic circulation
The arrangement of the **splanchnic circulation** (liver and digestive organs) is a partial exception to the parallel organization of the systemic vasculature (see Figure 1). Although a fraction of the blood supply to the liver is provided by the hepatic artery, the liver receives most (approximately 70%) of its blood via the **portal vein**. This vessel carries venous blood that has passed through the capillary beds of the stomach, spleen, pancreas and intestine. Most of the liver's circulation is therefore *in series* with that of the digestive organs. This arrangement facilitates hepatic uptake of nutrients and detoxification of foreign substances that have been absorbed during digestion. This type of sequential perfusion of two capillary beds is referred to as a **portal circulation**. A somewhat different type of portal circulation is also found within the kidney.

The lymphatic system
The body contains a parallel circulatory system of **lymphatic vessels** and **nodes** (see Chapter 20). The lymphatic system functions to return to the cardiovascular system the approximately 8 L/day of interstitial fluid that leaves the exchange vessels to enter body tissues. The larger lymphatic vessels pass through nodes containing lymphocytes, which act to mount an immune response to microbes, bacterial toxins and other foreign material carried into the lymphatic system with the interstitial fluid.

4 Vascular histology and smooth muscle cell ultrastructure

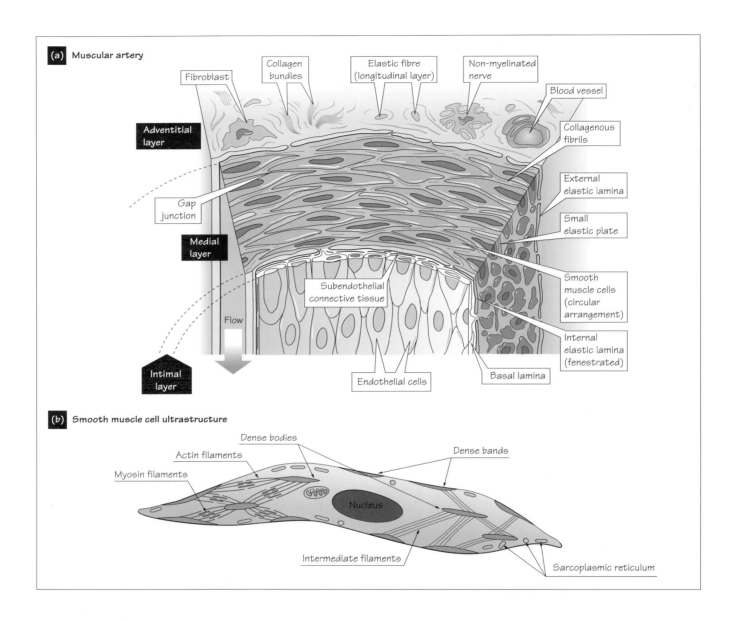

(a) Muscular artery

Fibroblast · Collagen bundles · Elastic fibre (longitudinal layer) · Non-myelinated nerve · Blood vessel · Collagenous fibrils · External elastic lamina · Small elastic plate · Smooth muscle cells (circular arrangement) · Internal elastic lamina (fenestrated) · Basal lamina · Endothelial cells · Subendothelial connective tissue · Flow · Intimal layer · Medial layer · Gap junction · Adventitial layer

(b) Smooth muscle cell ultrastructure

Dense bodies · Actin filaments · Dense bands · Myosin filaments · Nucleus · Intermediate filaments · Sarcoplasmic reticulum

Larger blood vessels share a common three-layered structure. Figure 4a illustrates the arrangement of these layers, or *tunics*, in a muscular artery.

A thin inner layer, the **tunica intima**, comprises an endothelial cell monolayer (**endothelium**) supported by connective tissue. The endothelial cells lining the vascular lumen are sealed to each other by tight **junctions**, which restrict the diffusion of large molecules across the endothelium. The endothelial cells have a crucial role in controlling vascular permeability, vasoconstriction, angiogenesis (growth of new blood vessels) and regulation of haemostasis.

The intima is relatively thicker in larger arteries, and contains some smooth muscle cells in large and medium-sized arteries and veins.

The thick middle layer, the **tunica media**, is separated from the intima by a fenestrated (perforated) sheath, the **internal elastic lamina**, mostly composed of elastin. The media contains **smooth muscle cells** embedded in an **extracellular matrix** (ECM) composed mainly of collagen, elastin and proteoglycans. The cells are shaped like elongated and irregular spindles or cylinders with tapering ends, and are 15–100 μm long. In the arterial system, they are

The Cardiovascular System at a Glance, Fourth Edition. Philip I. Aaronson, Jeremy P.T. Ward, and Michelle J. Connolly.

orientated circularly or in a low-pitch spiral, so that the vascular lumen narrows when they contract. Individual cells are long enough to wrap around small arterioles several times.

Adjacent smooth muscle cells form **gap junctions**. These are areas of close cellular contact in which arrays of large channels called **connexons** span both cell membranes, allowing ions to flow from one cell to another. The smooth muscle cells therefore form a **syncytium**, in which depolarization spreads from each cell to its neighbours.

An **external elastic lamina** separates the tunica media from the outer layer, the **tunica adventitia**. This contains collagenous tissue supporting fibroblasts and nerves. In large arteries and veins, the adventitia contains **vasa vasorum**, small blood vessels that also penetrate into the outer portion of the media and supply the vascular wall with oxygen and nutrients.

These three layers are also present in the venous system, but are less distinct. Compared with arteries, veins have a thinner tunica media containing a smaller amount of smooth muscle cells, which also tend to have a more random orientation.

The protein **elastin** is found mainly in the arteries. Molecules of elastin are arranged into a network of randomly coiled fibres. These molecular 'springs' allow arteries to expand during systole and then rebound during diastole to keep the blood flowing forward. This is particularly important in the aorta and other large elastic arteries, in which the media contains fenestrated sheets of elastin separating the smooth muscle cells into multiple concentric layers (lamellae).

The fibrous protein **collagen** is present in all three layers of the vascular wall, and functions as a framework that anchors the smooth muscle cells in place. At high internal pressures, the collagen network becomes very rigid, limiting vascular distensibility. This is particularly important in veins, which have a higher collagen content than arteries.

Exchange vessel structure

Capillaries and postcapillary venules are tubes formed of a single layer of overlapping endothelial cells. This is supported and surrounded on the external side by the **basal lamina**, a 50–100 nm layer of fibrous proteins including collagen, and glycoproteins. **Pericytes**, isolated cells that can give rise to smooth muscle cells during angiogenesis, adhere to the outside of the basal lamina, especially in postcapillary venules. The luminal side of the endothelium is coated by **glycocalyx**, a dense glycoprotein network attached to the cell membrane.

There are three types of capillaries, and these differ in their locations and permeabilities. Their structures are illustrated in Chapter 20.

Continuous capillaries occur in skin, muscles, lungs and the central nervous system. They have a low permeability to molecules that cannot pass readily through cell membranes, owing to the presence of tight junctions which bring the overlapping membranes of adjacent endothelial cells into close contact. The tight junctions run around the perimeter of each cell, forming a seal restricting the paracellular flow of molecules of molecular weight (MW) >10 000. These junctions are especially tight in most capillaries of the central nervous system, and form an integral part of the **blood–brain barrier** (see Chapter 20).

Fenestrated capillaries are much more permeable than continuous capillaries. These are found in endocrine glands, renal glomeruli, intestinal villi and other tissues in which large amounts of fluid or metabolites enter or leave capillaries. In addition to having leakier intercellular junctions, the endothelial cells of these capillaries contain **fenestrae**, circular pores of diameter 50–100 nm spanning areas of the cells where the cytoplasm is thinned. Except in the renal glomeruli, fenestrae are usually covered by a thin perforated diaphragm.

Discontinuous capillaries or **sinusoids** are found in liver, spleen and bone marrow. These are large, irregularly shaped capillaries with gaps between the endothelial cells wide enough to allow large proteins and even erythrocytes to cross the capillary wall.

Smooth muscle cell ultrastructure

The cytoplasm of vascular smooth muscle cells contains thin **actin** and thick **myosin** filaments (Figure 4b). Instead of being aligned into sarcomeres as in cardiac myocytes, groups of actin filaments running roughly parallel to the long axis of the cell are anchored at one end into elongated **dense bodies** in the cytoplasm and **dense bands** along the inner face of the cell membrane. Dense bodies and bands are linked by bundles of **intermediate filaments** composed mainly of the proteins **desmin** and **vimentin** to form the **cytoskeleton**, an internal scaffold giving the cell its shape. The free ends of the actin filaments interdigitate with myosin filaments. The myosin crossbridges are structured so that the actin filaments on either side of a myosin filament are pulled in opposite directions during crossbridge cycling. This draws the dense bodies towards each other, causing the cytoskeleton, and therefore the cell, to shorten. The dense bands are attached to the ECM by membrane-spanning proteins called **integrins**, allowing force development to be distributed throughout the vascular wall. The interaction between the ECM and integrins is a dynamic process which is affected by forces exerted on the matrix by the pressure inside the vessel. This allows the integrins, which are signalling molecules capable of influencing both cytoskeletal structure and signal transduction, to orchestrate cellular responses to changes in pressure.

The **sarcoplasmic reticulum** (SR, also termed smooth endoplasmic reticulum) occupies 2–6% of cell volume. This network of tubes and flattened sacs permeates the cell and contains a high concentration (~0.5 mmol/L) of free Ca^{2+}. Elements of the SR closely approach the cell membrane. Several types of Ca^{2+}-regulated ion channels and transporters are concentrated in these areas of the plasmalemma, which may have an important role in cellular excitation.

The nucleus is located in the central part of the cell. Organelles including rough endoplasmic reticulum, Golgi complex and mitochondria are mainly found in the perinuclear region.

5 Constituents of blood

Blood cells

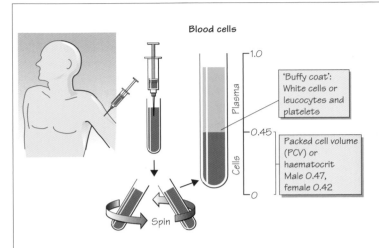

'Buffy coat': White cells or leucocytes and platelets

Packed cell volume (PCV) or haematocrit
Male 0.47, female 0.42

Spin

Composition of plasma

		Normal range	Units
Osmolality		280–295	mosm/kg H_2O
Electrolytes			
Na^+		135–145	mmol/L
K^+		3.5–5.0	mmol/L
Ca^{2+}	Total	2.2–2.6	mmol/L
	~50% Free	1.0–1.3	mmol/L
Mg^{2+}	Total	0.7–1.1	
	~50% Free	0.3–0.6	mmol/L
Cl^-		98–108	
HCO_3^-		22–30	mmol/L
Inorganic phosphate ~85–90% Free		0.8–1.4	mmol/L
Proteins (−ve charge)		~14	mmol/L
Cells			
Erythrocytes	male	4.7–6.1	$\times 10^{-12}$/L
	female	4.2–5.4	
Packed Cell Volume (PCV)	male	0.41–0.52	(no unit)
(Haematocrit)	female	0.36–0.48	
Haemoglobin (Hb)	male	130–180	g/L
	female	120–160	
Leucocytes (total) (White blood cell count, WBCC)		4–11	$\times 10^9$/L
Platelets		150–400	$\times 10^9$/L

Erythrocytes (red cells)

Approximate cell diameter $= 6.5–8.8\mu m$

Mean cell volume (**MCV**) $= \dfrac{PCV}{RCC} = $ ~85fL (85×10^{-15}L)

Mean cell haemoglobin (**MCH**) $= \dfrac{Hb}{RCC} = $ ~30pg (30×10^{-12}g)

Mean cell haemoglobin concentration (**MCHC**) $= \dfrac{MCH}{MCV}$ or $\dfrac{Hb}{PCV} = $ ~350g/L

Relative proportions of leucocytes (total count ~ 4–11 x 10^9 per litre)

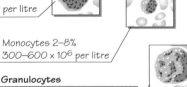
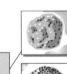
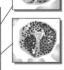

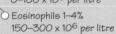

Lymphocytes 20–40%
1500–3000 x 10^6 per litre

Monocytes 2–8%
300–600 x 10^6 per litre

Granulocytes

Basophils ~0.5%
0–100 x 10^6 per litre

Eosinophils 1–4%
150–300 x 10^6 per litre

Neutrophils 50–70%
3000–6000 x 10^6 per litre

Protein composition of plasma

	Average plasma concentration (g/L)	Molecular weight (x 1000)	Functions include
Albumin	48.0	69	Colloidal osmotic pressure; binds hormones, drugs, etc.
α-globulins	5.5	16–90	Copper transport, binds haemoglobin, antiprotease
β-globulins			
Transferrin	3.0	90	Iron transport
Prothrombin	1.0	68	Haemostasis
Plasminogen	0.7	140	Haemostasis
Components of complement	1.6	~200	Immune system
Fibrinogen	3.0	350	Haemostasis
γ-globulins	13.0	150–200 (IgM, 1000)	Immunoglobulins (mostly IgG)

The Cardiovascular System at a Glance, Fourth Edition. Philip I. Aaronson, Jeremy P.T. Ward, and Michelle J. Connolly.

The primary function of blood is to deliver O_2 and energy sources to the tissues, and to remove CO_2 and waste products. It contains elements of the defence and immune systems, is important for regulation of temperature and transports hormones and other signalling molecules between tissues. In a 70-kg man blood volume is ~5500 mL, or 8% of body weight. Blood consists of **plasma** and **blood cells**. If blood is centrifuged, the cells sediment as the **packed cell volume** (PCV, haematocrit), normally ~45% of total volume (i.e. PCV = 0.45) in men, less in women (Figure 5).

Plasma

The plasma volume is ~5% of body weight. It consists of ions in solution and a variety of plasma proteins. Normal ranges for key constituents are shown in Figure 5. After clotting, a straw-coloured fluid called **serum** remains, from which fibrinogen and other clotting factors have been removed. The relative osmotic pressures of plasma, interstitial and intracellular fluid are critical for maintenance of tissue cell volume, and are related to the amount of osmotically active particles (molecules) per litre, or **osmolarity** (mosmol/L); as plasma is not an ideal fluid (it contains slow diffusing proteins), the term **osmolality** (mosmol/kg H_2O) is often used instead. Plasma **osmolality** is ~290 mosmol/kg H_2O, mostly due to dissolved ions and small diffusible molecules (e.g. glucose and urea). These diffuse easily across capillaries, and the **crystalloid osmotic pressure** they exert is therefore the same either side of the capillary wall. Proteins do not easily pass through capillary walls, and are responsible for the **oncotic** (or colloidal osmotic) pressure of the plasma. This is much smaller than crystalloid osmotic pressure, but is critical for fluid transfer across capillary walls because it differs between plasma and interstitial fluid (see Chapter 21). Oncotic pressure is expressed in terms of pressure, and in plasma is normally ~25 mmHg. Maintenance of plasma osmolality is vital for regulation of blood volume (see Chapter 29).

Ionic composition

Na^+ is the most prevalent ion in plasma, and the main determinant of plasma osmolality. The figure shows concentrations of the major ions; others are present in smaller amounts. Changes in ionic concentration can have major consequences for excitable tissues (e.g. K^+, Ca^{2+}). Whereas Na^+, K^+ and Cl^- completely dissociate in plasma, Ca^{2+} and Mg^{2+} are partly bound to plasma proteins, so that free concentration is ~50% of the total.

Proteins

Normal total plasma protein concentration is 65–83 g/L. Most plasma proteins other than γ-globulins (see below) are synthesized in the liver. Proteins can ionize as either acids or bases because they have both NH_2 and COOH groups. At pH 7.4 they are mostly in the anionic (acidic) form. Their ability to accept or donate H^+ means they can act as buffers, and account for ~15% of the buffering capacity of blood. Plasma proteins have important transport functions. They bind with many hormones (e.g. cortisol, thyroxine), metals (e.g. iron) and drugs, and therefore modulate their free concentration and thus biological activity. Plasma proteins encompass **albumin**, **fibrinogen** and **globulins** (Figure 5). Globulins are further classified as α-, β- and γ-globulins. β-Globulins include transferrin (iron transport), components of complement (immune system), and prothrombin and plasminogen, which with fibrinogen are involved in blood clotting (Chapter 7). The most important γ-globulins are the immunoglobulins (e.g. IgG, IgE, IgM).

Blood cells

In the adult, all blood cells are produced in the **red bone marrow**, although in the fetus, and following bone marrow damage in the adult, they are also produced in the liver and spleen. The marrow contains a small number of **uncommitted stem cells**, which differentiate into specific **committed stem cells** for each blood cell type. **Platelets** are not true cells, but small (~3 μm) vesicle-like structures formed from **megakaryocytes** in the bone marrow, containing clearly visible **dense granules**. Platelets play a key role in haemostasis (Chapter 7), and have a lifespan of ~4 days.

Erythrocytes

Erythrocytes (red cells) are by far the most numerous cells in the blood (Figure 5), with ~5.5×10^{12}/L in males (red cell count, RCC). Erythrocytes are biconcave discs with no nucleus, and a mean cell volume (**MCV**) of ~85 fL. Each contains ~30 pg haemoglobin (mean cell haemoglobin, **MCH**), which is responsible for carriage of O_2 and plays an important part in acid–base buffering. Blood contains ~160 g/L (male) and ~140 g/L (female) haemoglobin. The shape and flexibility of erythrocytes allows them to deform easily and pass through the capillaries. When blood is allowed to stand in the presence of anticoagulant, the cells slowly sediment (erythrocyte sedimentation rate, **ESR**). The ESR is increased when cells stack together (form *rouleaux*), and in pregnancy and inflammatory disease, and decreased by low plasma fibrinogen. Erythrocytes have an average lifespan of 120 days. Their formation (erythropoiesis) and related diseases are discussed in Chapter 6.

Leucocytes (white cells) and platelets

Leucocytes defend the body against infection by foreign material. The normal white blood cell count (WBCC, see Figure 5) increases greatly in disease (**leucocytosis**). In the newborn infant the WBCC is ~20×10^9/L. Three main types are present in blood: **granulocytes** (polymorphonuclear leucocytes, PMN), **lymphocytes** and **monocytes**. Granulocytes are further classified as **neutrophils** (containing neutral-staining granules), **eosinophils** (acid-staining granules) and **basophils** (basic-staining granules). All contribute to inflammation by releasing mediators (cytokines) when activated.

Neutrophils have a key role in the innate immune system, and migrate to areas of infection (**chemotaxis**) within minutes, where they destroy bacteria by **phagocytosis**. They are a major constituent of pus. They have a half-life of ~6 h in blood, days in tissue. *Eosinophils* are less motile and longer lived, and phagocytose larger parasites. They increase in allergic reactions, and contribute to allergic disease (e.g. asthma) by release of pro-inflammatory cytokines. *Basophils* release histamine and heparin as part of the inflammatory response, and are similar to tissue **mast** cells. *Lymphocytes* originate in the marrow but mature in the lymph nodes, thymus and spleen before returning to the circulation. Most remain in the lymphatic system. Lymphocytes are critical components of the **immune** system and are of three main forms: B cells which produce immunoglobulins (antibodies), T cells which coordinate the immune response, and natural killer (NK) cells which kill infected or cancerous cells.

Monocytes are phagocytes with a clear cytoplasm and are larger and longer lived than granulocytes. After formation in the marrow they circulate in the blood for ~72 h before entering the tissues to become **macrophages**, which unlike granulocytes can also dispose of dead cell debris. Macrophages form the **reticuloendothelial system** in liver, spleen and lymph nodes.

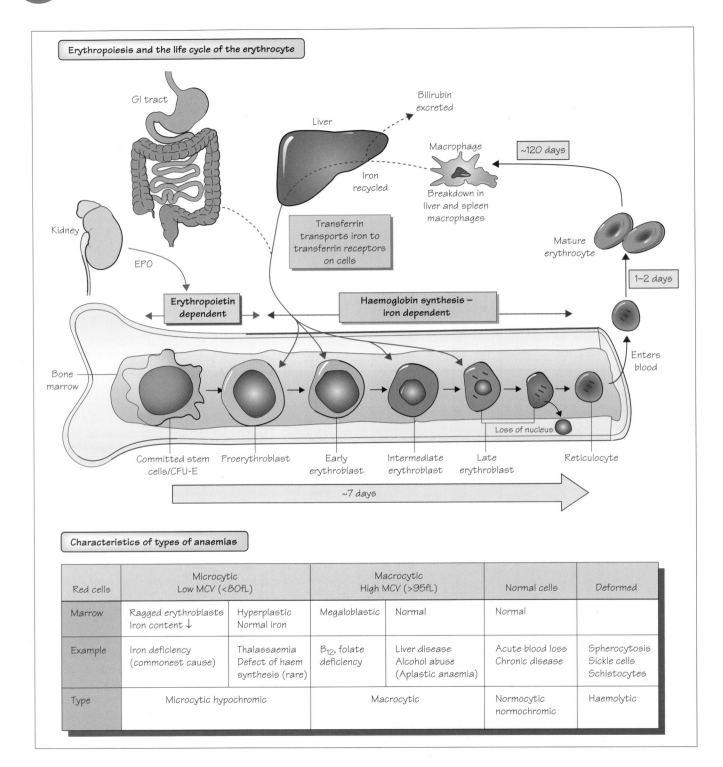

Erythropoiesis and the life cycle of the erythrocyte

GI tract

Liver

Bilirubin excreted

Macrophage

~120 days

Iron recycled

Breakdown in liver and spleen macrophages

Transferrin transports iron to transferrin receptors on cells

Mature erythrocyte

Kidney

EPO

Erythropoietin dependent

Haemoglobin synthesis – iron dependent

1–2 days

Enters blood

Bone marrow

Loss of nucleus

Committed stem cells/CFU-E | Proerythroblast | Early erythroblast | Intermediate erythroblast | Late erythroblast | Reticulocyte

~7 days

Characteristics of types of anaemias

Red cells	Microcytic Low MCV (<80fL)		Macrocytic High MCV (>95fL)		Normal cells	Deformed
Marrow	Ragged erythroblasts Iron content ↓	Hyperplastic Normal iron	Megaloblastic	Normal	Normal	
Example	Iron deficiency (commonest cause)	Thalassaemia Defect of haem synthesis (rare)	B_{12}, folate deficiency	Liver disease Alcohol abuse (Aplastic anaemia)	Acute blood loss Chronic disease	Spherocytosis Sickle cells Schistocytes
Type	Microcytic hypochromic		Macrocytic		Normocytic normochromic	Haemolytic

Erythropoiesis

Erythropoiesis, the formation of red cells (erythrocytes), occurs in the red bone marrow of adults and the liver and spleen of the fetus. It can also occur in the liver and spleen of adults following bone marrow damage. Erythropoiesis is primarily controlled by **erythropoietin**, a glycoprotein hormone secreted primarily by the kidneys in response to hypoxia; about 10–15% is produced by the liver, the major source for the fetus. Other factors such as corticosteroids and growth hormones can also stimulate erythropoiesis.

The Cardiovascular System at a Glance, Fourth Edition. Philip I. Aaronson, Jeremy P.T. Ward, and Michelle J. Connolly.

Erythropoiesis begins when uncommitted stem cells commit to the erythrocyte lineage and under the influence of erythropoietin transform into rapidly growing precursor cells (colony forming unit erythroid cells, CFU-E) and then **proerythroblasts** (Figure 6). These large cells are packed with ribosomes, and it is here that haemoglobin synthesis begins. Development and maturation proceeds through early (basophilic), intermediate (polychromatic) and finally late (orthochromatic) **erythroblasts** (or normoblasts) of decreasing size. As cell division ceases, ribosomal content decreases and haemoglobin increases. The late erythroblast finally loses its nucleus to become a **reticulocyte**, a young erythrocyte still retaining the vestiges of a ribosomal reticulum. Reticulocytes enter the blood and, as they age, the reticulum disappears and the characteristic biconcave shape develops. About 2×10^{11} erythrocytes are produced from the marrow each day, and normally 1–2% of circulating red cells are reticulocytes. This increases when erythropoiesis is enhanced, for example by increased **erythropoietin** due to hypoxia associated with respiratory disease or altitude. This can greatly increase erythrocyte numbers (**polycythaemia**) and haematocrit. Conversely, erythropoietin levels may fall in kidney disease, chronic inflammation and liver cirrhosis, resulting in anaemia.

Erythrocytes are destroyed by **macrophages** in the liver and spleen after ~120 days. The spleen also sequesters and eradicates defective erythrocytes. The haem group is split from haemoglobin and converted to **biliverdin** and then **bilirubin**. The iron is conserved and recycled via **transferrin**, an iron transport protein, or stored in **ferritin**. Bilirubin is a brown–yellow compound that is excreted in the bile. An increased rate of haemoglobin breakdown results in excess bilirubin, which stains the tissues (**jaundice**).

Haemoglobin

Haemoglobin has four subunits, each containing a polypeptide **globin** chain and an iron-containing porphyrin, **haem**, which are synthesized separately. Haem is synthesized from succinic acid and glycine in the mitochondria, and contains one atom of iron in the **ferrous** state (Fe^{2+}). One molecule of haemoglobin has therefore four atoms of iron, and binds four molecules of O_2. There are several types of haemoglobin, relating to the globin chains; the haem moiety is unchanged. Adult haemoglobin (Hb A) has two α and two β chains. Fetal haemoglobin (Hb F) has two γ chains in place of the β chains, and a high affinity for O_2. **Haemoglobinopathies** are due to abnormal haemoglobins.

Sickle cell anaemia occurs in 10% of the Black population, and is caused by substitution of a glutamic acid by valine in the β chain; this haemoglobin is called Hb S. At a low Po_2 Hb S gels, causing deformation (*sickling*) of the erythrocyte. The cell is less flexible and prone to fragmentation, and there is an increased rate of breakdown by macrophages. Heterozygous patients with less than 40% Hb S normally have no symptoms (**sickle cell trait**). Homozygous patients with more than 70% Hb S develop full **sickle cell anaemia**, with acute episodes of pain resulting from blockage of blood vessels, congestion of liver and spleen with red cells, and leg ulcers.

Thalassaemia involves defective synthesis of α- or β-globin chains. Several genes are involved. In β thalassaemia there are fewer or no β chains available, so α chains bind to γ (Hb F) or δ chains (Hb A_2). Thalassaemia major (severe β thalassaemia) causes severe anaemia, and regular transfusions are required, leading to iron overload. In heterozygous β thalassaemia minor there are no symptoms, although erythrocytes are **microcytic** and **hypochromic**, i.e. **mean cell volume** (MCV), **mean cell haemoglobin content** (MCH) and **mean cell haemoglobin concentration** (MCHC) are reduced. In α **thalassaemia** there are fewer or no α chains. In the latter case haemoglobin does not bind O_2, and infants do not survive (**hydrops fetalis**). When some α chains are present, patients surviving as adults may produce some Hb H (four β chains); this precipitates in the red cells which are then destroyed in the spleen.

Anaemia

Blood loss (e.g. haemorrhage, heavy menstruation) or chronic disease (e.g. infection, tumours, renal failure) may simply reduce the number of erythrocytes. When these have a normal MCV and MCH (see Chapter 5), this is termed **normocytic normochromic** anaemia.

Iron deficiency is the most common cause of anemia. The dietary requirement for iron is small, as the body has an efficient recycling system, but is increased with significant blood loss. Women have a higher requirement for dietary iron than men because of menstruation, and also during pregnancy. Iron deficiency causes defective haemoglobin formation and a **microcytic hypochromic** anaemia (reduced MCV and MCH).

Vitamin B_{12} (cobalamin) and folate are required for maturation of erythroblasts, and deficiencies of either cause **megaloblastic anaemia**. The erythroblasts are unusually large (megaloblasts), and mature as erythrocytes with a high MCV and MCH, although MCHC is normal. Erythrocyte numbers are greatly reduced, and rate of destruction increased. Folate deficiency is mostly related to poor diet, particularly in the elderly or poor; folate is commonly given with iron during pregnancy. Alcoholism and some anticonvulsant drugs (e.g. phenytoin) impairs folate utilization. **Pernicious anaemia** is caused by defective absorption of vitamin B_{12} from the gut, where it is transported as a complex with intrinsic factor produced by the gastric mucosa. Damage to the latter results in pernicious anaemia. B_{12} deficiency can also occur in strict vegans.

Aplastic anaemia results from aplastic (non-functional) bone marrow and causes **pancytopenia** (reduced red, white and platelet cell count). It is dangerous but uncommon. It can be caused by drugs (particularly anticancer), radiation, infections (e.g. viral hepatitis, TB) and pregnancy, where it has a 90% mortality. A rare inherited condition, **Fanconi's anaemia**, involves defective stem cell production and differentiation.

Haemolytic anaemia involves an excessive rate of erythrocyte destruction, and thus causes jaundice. Causes include blood transfusion mismatch, **haemolytic anaemia of the newborn** (see Chapter 9), abnormal erythrocyte fragility and haemoglobins, and autoimmune, liver and hereditary diseases. In **hereditary haemolytic anaemia** (familial spherocytosis) erythrocytes are more spheroid and fragile, and are rapidly destroyed in the spleen. It is relatively common, affecting 1 in 5000 Caucasians. Jaundice is common at birth but may appear after several years. Aplastic anaemia may occur after infections, and megaloblastic anaemia from folate deficiency as a result of high bone marrow activity.

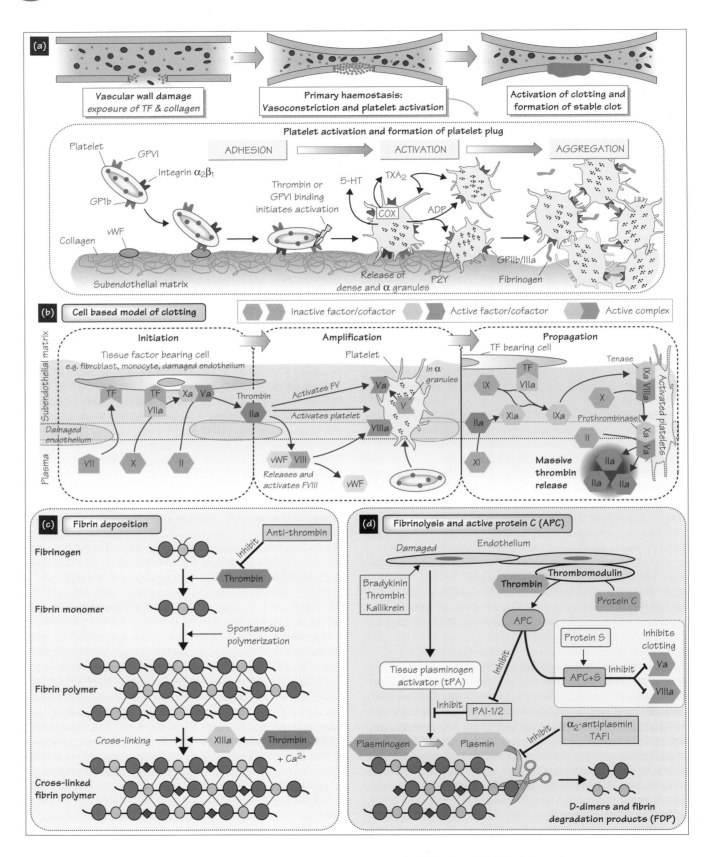

The Cardiovascular System at a Glance, Fourth Edition. Philip I. Aaronson, Jeremy P.T. Ward, and Michelle J. Connolly.

Primary haemostasis (Figure 7a)

The immediate response to damage of the blood vessel wall is vasoconstriction, which reduces blood flow. This is followed by a sequence of events leading to sealing of the wound by a clot. Collagen in the exposed subendothelial matrix binds **von Willebrand factor** (vWF), which in turn binds to glycoprotein Ib (**GPIb**) receptors on platelets, the first stage of **platelet adhesion**. This initial tethering promotes binding of platelet **integrin $\alpha_2\beta_1$** and **GPVI** receptors directly to collagen. Binding of receptors initiates **activation**, partly by increasing intracellular Ca^{2+}. Platelets change shape, put out pseudopodia and make thromboxane A_2 (**TXA$_2$**) via cyclooxygenase (**COX**). TXA$_2$ releases mediators from platelet **dense granules**, including **serotonin** (5-HT) and adenosine diphosphate (**ADP**), and from α **granules** vWF, factor V (see below) and agents that promote vascular repair. TXA$_2$ and 5-HT also promote vasoconstriction. ADP activates more platelets via **P2Y$_{12}$** purinergic receptors, causing activation of **fibrinogen** (GPIIb/IIIa) receptors and exposure of **phospholipid** (PLD) on the platelet surface. Plasma fibrinogen binds to GPIIb/IIIa receptors causing the platelets to **aggregate** (stick together) forming a soft **platelet plug** (Figure 7a). This is stabilized with **fibrin** during clotting. Note that **thrombin** (see below) is also a potent platelet activator.

Formation of the blood clot (Figures 7b,c)

The final stage of blood clotting (coagulation) is formation of the clot – a tight mesh of **fibrin** entrapping platelets and blood cells. The process is complex, involving sequential conversion of proenzymes to active enzymes (**factors**; e.g. factor X → Xa). The ultimate purpose is to produce a massive burst of **thrombin** (factor IIa), a protease that cleaves fibrinogen to fibrin. The **cell-based model** of clotting (Figure 7b) has replaced the older extrinsic and intrinsic pathways. Most of the action in this model occurs on the cell surface (hence its name).

The **initial phase** of clotting is initiated when cells in the subendothelial matrix that bear **tissue factor** (TF; thromboplastin) are exposed to factor VIIa from plasma. Such cells include fibroblasts and monocytes, but damaged endothelium and circulating cell fragments containing TF (microparticles) can also initiate clotting. TF forms a complex with factor VIIa (**TF:VIIa**) which activates **factor X** (and IX, see below). **Factor Xa** with its cofactor Va then converts **prothrombin** (factor II) to thrombin; activation of both factor X and prothrombin require Ca^{2+}. Comparatively little thrombin is produced at this time, but sufficient to initiate the **amplification phase**. Activity of these processes is normally suppressed by tissue factor pathway inhibitor (**TFPI**), which inhibits and forms a complex with factor Xa, which then inhibits TF:VIIa; however, the influx of plasma factors after damage overwhelms this suppression.

The **amplification phase** (sometimes viewed as part of the propagation phase) takes place on platelets (Figure 7b). Thrombin produced in the initial phase activates further platelets, and membrane-bound factor V which is released from platelet α granules. Factor VIII is normally bound to circulating vWF, which protects it from degradation. Thrombin cleaves factor VIII from vWF and activates it, when it binds to the platelet membrane.

The scene is now set for the **propagation phase**. Either factor XIa (itself activated by thrombin) or TF:VIIa can activate factor IX, which binds and forms a complex with factor VIIIa on the platelet membrane called **tenase**; this is a much more powerful activator of factor X than TF:VIIa. Factors Xa and Va then bind to form **prothrombinase** on the platelet membrane. This process leads to a massive burst of thrombin production, 1000-fold greater than in the initial phase and localized to activated platelets.

Factor XII (Hageman factor, not shown) is probably of limited significance, as deficiency does not lead to bleeding. It is activated by negative charge on glass and collagen, and can activate factor XI. It may be involved in pathological clotting in the brain.

Thrombin cleaves small fibrinopeptides from fibrinogen to form fibrin monomers (Figure 7c), which spontaneously **polymerize**. This polymer is **cross-linked** by **factor XIIIa** (activated by thrombin in the presence of Ca^{2+}) to create a tough network of fibrin fibres and a **stable clot**. Retraction of entrapped platelets contracts the clot by ~60%, making it tougher and assisting repair by drawing the edges of the wound together.

Inhibitors of haemostasis and fibrinolysis

Inhibitory mechanisms are vital to prevent inappropriate clotting (**thrombosis**). **Prostacyclin** (PGI$_2$) and nitric oxide from undamaged endothelium impede platelet adhesion and activation. **Antithrombin** inhibits thrombin, factor Xa and IXa/tenase; its activity is strongly potentiated by **heparin**, a polysaccharide. *Heparan* on endothelial cells is similar. **TFPI** has already been mentioned. **Thrombomodulin** on endothelial cells binds thrombin and prevents it cleaving fibrinogen; instead, it activates **protein C** (APC) which with its cofactor **protein S** inactivates cofactors Va and VIIIa, and hence tenase and prothrombinase (Figure 7d).

Fibrinolysis is the process by which a clot is broken down by **plasmin**, a protease (Figure 7d). This creates soluble fibrin degradation products (**FDPs**) including small **D-dimers**. Plasmin is formed from fibrin-bound **plasminogen** by tissue plasminogen activator (**tPA**), released from damaged endothelial cells in response to bradykinin, thrombin and kallikrein. **Urokinase** (uPA) is similar. APC inactivates an inhibitor of plasminogen activator inhibitor (tPA; **PAI-1** and 2), and so promotes fibrinolysis (Figure 7d). Plasmin is itself inactivated by α_2-**antiplasmin**, and inhibited by thrombin activated fibrinolysis inhibitor (**TAFI**).

Defects in haemostasis

The most common hereditary disorder is **haemophilia A**, a deficiency of factor VIII sex linked to males. **Christmas disease** is a deficiency of factor IX, and **von Willebrand disease** a deficiency of vWF. The latter leads to defective platelet adhesion and reduced availability of factor VIII, which is stabilized by vWF. The liver requires **vitamin K** for correct synthesis of prothrombin and factors VII, IX and X. As vitamin K is obtained from intestinal bacteria and food, disorders of fat absorption or liver disease can result in deficiency and defective clotting. **Factor V Leiden** is brought about by a mutant factor V that cannot be inactivated by APC. Five per cent carry the gene, which causes a fivefold increase in the risk of thrombosis. **Antiphospholipid syndrome** is caused by phospholipid-binding antibodies (e.g. cardiolipin, lupus anticoagulant) which may inhibit APC and protein S, or facilitate cleavage of prothrombin. It is associated with recurrent thrombosis and linked to 20% of strokes in people under 50 years, more common in females.

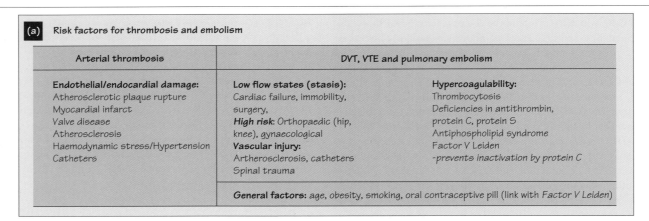

(a) Risk factors for thrombosis and embolism

Arterial thrombosis	DVT, VTE and pulmonary embolism	
Endothelial/endocardial damage: Atherosclerotic plaque rupture, Myocardial infarct, Valve disease, Atherosclerosis, Haemodynamic stress/Hypertension, Catheters	**Low flow states (stasis):** Cardiac failure, immobility, surgery, **High risk:** Orthopaedic (hip, knee), gynaecological **Vascular injury:** Artherosclerosis, catheters Spinal trauma	**Hypercoagulability:** Thrombocytosis, Deficiencies in antithrombin, protein C, protein S, Antiphospholipid syndrome, Factor V Leiden, -prevents inactivation by protein C
	General factors: age, obesity, smoking, oral contraceptive pill (link with *Factor V Leiden*)	

(b) Antiplatelet drugs: action on platelet activation and aggregation

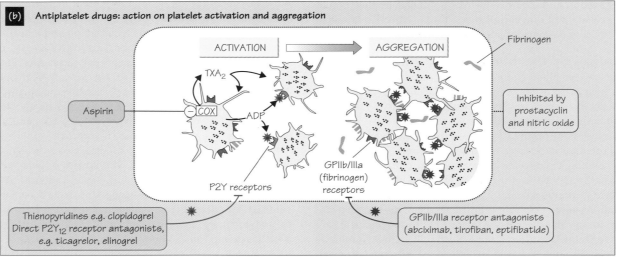

(c) Anticoagulant drugs: action on clotting cascade

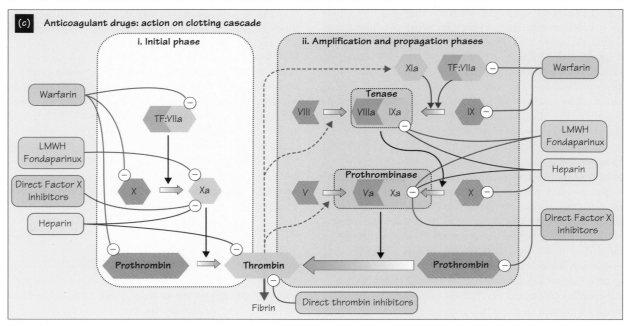

The Cardiovascular System at a Glance, Fourth Edition. Philip I. Aaronson, Jeremy P.T. Ward, and Michelle J. Connolly.
© 2013 John Wiley & Sons, Ltd. Published 2013 by John Wiley & Sons, Ltd.

Thrombosis

Thrombosis and embolism are ultimately the main cause of death in the industrialized world. Thrombosis is inappropriate activation of haemostasis, with clots (**thrombi**) forming inside blood vessels. If thrombi fragment they can be carried in the blood as **emboli**, and block downstream blood vessels causing infarction. Most commonly fatalities are due to thrombosis as a result of **atherosclerotic plaque rupture** in acute coronary syndromes (see Chapter 42), or venous thromboembolism (**VTE**), particularly **pulmonary embolism**, following **deep vein thrombosis (DVT)**. **Virchow's triad** of *endothelial damage, blood stasis* and *hypercoagulability* predispose to thrombosis. Endothelial (or endocardial) damage is the most common cause of arterial thrombosis. Stasis (poor flow), which allows clotting factors to accumulate and unimpeded formation of thrombi, is the most common cause of DVT and VTE. **Risk factors** are shown in Figure 8a. Once formed, thrombi can undergo **dissolution** by fibrinolysis, **propagation** by accumulation of more fibrin and platelets, or **organization** with invasion of endothelial or smooth muscle cells and fibrosis. In **recanalization** channels form allowing blood to reflow. If not destroyed, thrombi may be incorporated into the vessel wall.

Arterial (white, platelet-rich) thrombi are primarily treated with antiplatelet drugs, while venous (red) thrombi are primarily treated with anticoagulants. All such therapies increase risk of bleeding, and may be contraindicated in patients with prior stroke, active ulcers, pregnancy or recent surgery.

Antiplatelet drugs (Figure 8b)

Aspirin (*acetylsalicylic acid*) is the most important antiplatelet drug. It irreversibly inhibits **cyclooxygenase (COX)**, the first enzyme in the sequence leading to formation of **thromboxane A_2** (**TXA_2**) and **prostacyclin (PGI_2)**. TXA_2 is produced by platelets and is a key platelet activator (see Chapter 7), whereas endothelium-derived PGI_2 inhibits platelet activation and aggregation. Because aspirin inhibits COX *irreversibly*, production of PGI_2 and TXA_2 only recovers when new COX is produced via gene transcription. This cannot occur in platelets, which lack nuclei (see Chapter 5), whereas endothelial cells make new COX within hours. Aspirin therapy therefore produces a sustained increase in the PGI_2:TXA_2 ratio, suppressing platelet activation and aggregation. Aspirin can cause gastrointestinal bleeding.

Thienopyridine derivatives such as **clopidogrel** indirectly and irreversibly block puringeric **P2Y receptors**, and thus ADP-induced platelet activation (see Chapter 7); however, they are prodrugs that require metabolism in the liver, and so take >24h for maximal effect. They are useful for aspirin-intolerant patients and preventing thrombi on coronary artery stents (see Chapter 42), and long-term treatment with clopidogrel plus aspirin is beneficial in acute coronary syndromes. New direct **$P2Y_{12}$ receptor antagonists** such as ticagrelor and elinogrel have advantages including rapidity of action, and are effective for acute coronary syndrome.

Small peptide glycoprotein receptor inhibitors (**GPI**) such as tirofiban and eptifibatide and the monoclonal antibody abciximab prevent fibrinogen binding to **GPIIb/IIIa receptors** on activated platelets, thus inhibiting aggregation (see Chapter 7). In patients with unstable angina or undergoing high-risk angioplasty, a GPI combined with aspirin and heparin reduces short-term mortality, and the need for urgent revascularization.

Anticoagulant drugs (Figure 8c)

Heparin, a mixture of mucopolysaccharides derived from mast cells, activates **antithrombin**, which inhibits thrombin and factors X, IX and XI (see Chapter 7). Heparin must bind to both thrombin and antithrombin for inhibition of thrombin, but only antithrombin for inhibition of factor X. *Unfractionated* heparin has a large variability of action and causes thrombocytopenia in some patients. **Low molecular weight heparins** (LMWHs) have largely replaced unfractionated heparin in clinical use, as they have a longer half-life and predictable dose responses; thrombocytopenia is rare. LMWHs only bind to antithrombin, and are therefore more effective at inhibiting factor X. They are given subcutaneously, and are first line drugs for routine thromboprophylaxis. **Fondaparinux** is a synthetic pentasaccharide that acts in a similar fashion to LMWH. **Bivalirudin** is a direct thrombin inhibitor delivered intravenously, with benefits of rapidity of action and reversal.

Warfarin (coumarin) is currently the most important oral anticoagulant. It inhibits vitamin K reductase, and thus γ-carboxylation of prothrombin and factors VII, IX and X in the liver; this prevents tethering to cells and hence activity (see Chapter 7). Warfarin is only effective *in vivo*. Although slow in onset (~1–2 days), it provides effective support for ~5 days. Numerous factors including disease and drugs affect the sensitivity to warfarin, so blood tests must be used routinely to monitor dosage, which is adjusted to give a **prothrombin time** international normalized ratio (**INR**) of ~3 (see below). Use of warfarin may decline following the advent of oral direct thrombin (e.g. **dabigatran**) and factor Xa antagonists (e.g. **rivaroxaban**). These have benefits of increased rapidity of action and reduced sensitivity to other drugs and disease, and a greatly reduced need for routine blood tests. Both are approved for prevention of VTE following hip and knee replacement surgery, and have been shown to be as effective as warfarin for prevention of atrial fibrillation-associated stroke.

Thrombolytic agents induce fibrinolysis by activating plasmin; tissue plasminogen activator (**tPA**) is the most important endogenous agent (see Chapter 7), and recombinant tPA the most commonly used clinically. Until relatively recently, thrombolysis was the recognized treatment for dissolution of life-threatening blood clots in coronary artery disease and acute MI, although with a severe risk of gut and intracerebral haemorrhage (stroke). It has now been largely replaced by emergency angioplasty – percutaneous coronary intervention (PCI) (see Chapter 43).

Some laboratory investigations

Prothrombin time (PT): time to clot formation following addition of thromboplastin (TF) (fibrinogen and Ca^{2+} in excess); normally ~14s. A measure of activity of vitamin K-dependent clotting factors, and thus important for titrating dose of **warfarin** (see above). It is expressed as **INR**, the ratio of the patient's PT to that of a standardized reference sample. INR is normally 1.

Activated partial thromboplastin time (aPTT): time to clot formation following addition of a surface activator (kaolin; activates factor XII), phospholipid and Ca^{2+} to plasma. Measures activity of factors in the amplification phase (i.e. not factor VIIa) (see Figure 7b). Normally 35–45s. Prolonged by relevant deficiencies.

D-dimers and fibrin degradation products (FDPs): indicative of fibrinolysis; raised in disseminated intravascular coagulation (**DIC**) and other thrombotic conditions. False positives common.

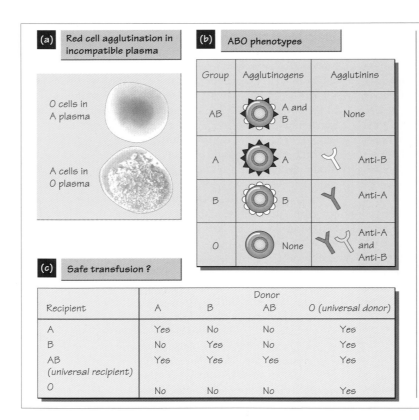

(a) **Red cell agglutination in incompatible plasma**

O cells in A plasma

A cells in O plasma

(b) **ABO phenotypes**

Group	Agglutinogens	Agglutinins
AB	A and B	None
A	A	Anti-B
B	B	Anti-A
O	None	Anti-A and Anti-B

(c) **Safe transfusion ?**

Recipient	Donor			
	A	B	AB	O (universal donor)
A	Yes	No	No	Yes
B	No	Yes	No	Yes
AB (universal recipient)	Yes	Yes	Yes	Yes
O	No	No	No	Yes

(d) **Relative distribution of ABO blood types by race**

Group	Caucasian	Far Eastern	Afro-Caribbean	Native American
A	41%	28%	28%	3%
B	10%	23%	20%	—
AB	4%	13%	5%	—
O	45%	36%	47%	97%

(e) **Distribution of Rhesus groups (Caucasians)**

Group	Proportion of population	Breakdown of genotypes
RH +	85%	35% DD 48% Dd 2% other + D
RH −	15%	.

Blood groups

If samples of blood from different individuals are mixed together, some combinations result in red cells sticking together as clumps (Figure 9a). This is called **agglutination**, and occurs when the **blood groups** are incompatible. It is caused when antigens (or **agglutinogens**) on the red cell membrane react with specific antibodies (or **agglutinins**) in the plasma. If the quantity (or **titre**) of antibodies is sufficiently high, they bind to their antigens on several red cells and glue the cells together, which then rupture (**haemolyse**). If this occurs following a blood transfusion it can lead to anaemia and other serious complications. The most important blood groups are the **ABO system** and **Rh (Rhesus)** groups.

The ABO system

The **ABO system** consists of four blood groups: A, B, AB and O. The precise group depends on the presence or absence of two antigens, A and B, on the red cells, and their respective antibodies, α and β, in the plasma (Figure 9b). The A and B antigens on red cells are mostly glycolipids that differ in respect of their terminal sugar. The antigens are also found as glycoproteins in other tissues, including salivary glands, pancreas, lungs and testes, and in saliva and semen.

Group A blood contains the A antigen and β antibody, and group B the B antigen and α antibody. Group AB has both A and B antigens, but neither antibody. Group O blood contains neither antigen, but both α and β antibodies. Group A blood cannot therefore be transfused into people of group B, or vice versa, because antibodies in the recipient react with their respective antigens on the donor red cells and cause agglutination (Figure 9c). As people of group AB have neither α nor β antibodies in the plasma, they can be transfused with blood from any group, and are called **universal recipients**. Group O red cells have neither antigen, and can therefore be transfused into any patient. People of group O are therefore called **universal donors**. Although group O blood contains both antibodies, this can normally be disregarded as they are diluted during transfusion and are bound and neutralized by free A or B antigens in the recipient's plasma. If large or repeated transfusions are required, blood of the same group is used.

Inheritance of ABO blood groups

The expression of A and B antigens is determined genetically. A and B allelomorphs (alternative gene types) are dominant, and O recessive. Therefore AO (**heterozygous**) and AA (**homozygous**)

The Cardiovascular System at a Glance, Fourth Edition. Philip I. Aaronson, Jeremy P.T. Ward, and Michelle J. Connolly.

genotypes both have group A phenotypes. An AB genotype produces both antigens, and is thus group AB. The proportion of each blood group varies according to race (Figure 9d), although group O is most common (35–50%). Native Americans are almost exclusively group O.

Rh groups

In ~85% of the population the red cells have a D antigen on the membrane (Figure 9e). Such people are called Rh+ (Rhesus positive), while those who lack the antigen are Rh– (Rhesus negative). Unlike ABO antigens, the D antigen is not found in other tissues. The antibody to D antigen (**anti-D agglutinin**) is not normally found in the plasma of Rh– individuals, but sensitization and subsequent antibody production occurs if a relatively small amount of Rh+ blood is introduced. This can result from transfusion, or when an Rh– mother has an Rh+ child, and fetal red blood cells enter the maternal circulation during birth. Occasionally, fetal cells may cross the placenta earlier in the pregnancy.

Inheritance of Rh groups

The gene corresponding to the D antigen is also called D, and is dominant. When D is absent from the chromosome, its place is taken by the allelomorph of D called d, which is recessive. Individuals who are homozygous and heterozygous for D will be Rh+. About 50% of the population are heterozygous for D, and ~35% homozygous. Blood typing for Rh groups is routinely performed for prospective parents to determine the likelihood of **haemolytic disease** in the offspring.

Haemolytic disease of the newborn

Most pregnancies with Rh– mothers and Rh+ fetuses are normal, but in some cases a severe reaction occurs. Anti-D antibody in the mother's blood can cross the placenta and agglutinate fetal red cells expressing D antigen. The titre of antibody is generally too low to be of consequence during a first pregnancy with a Rh+ fetus, but it can be dangerously increased during subsequent pregnancies, or if the mother was previously sensitized with Rh+ blood. Agglutination of the fetal red cells and consequent haemolysis can result in anaemia and other complications. This is known as **haemolytic disease of the newborn** or **erythroblastosis fetalis**. The haemoglobin released is broken down to bilirubin, which in excess results in **jaundice** (yellow staining of the tissues). If the degree of agglutination and anaemia is severe, the fetus develops severe jaundice and is grossly oedematous (**hydrops fetalis**), and often dies *in utero* or shortly after birth.

Prevention and treatment In previously unsensitized mothers, sensitization can be prevented by treatment with anti-D immunoglobulin after birth. This destroys any fetal Rh+ red cells in the maternal circulation before sensitization of the mother can occur. If haemolytic disease is evident in the fetus or newborn, the Rh+ blood can be replaced by Rh– blood immediately after birth. By the time the newborn infant has regenerated its own Rh+ red cells, the anti-D antibody from the mother will have been reduced to safe levels. Phototherapy is commonly used for jaundice, as light converts bilirubin to a more rapidly eliminated compound.

Other blood groups

Although there are other blood groups, these are of little clinical importance, as humans rarely develop antibodies to the respective antigens. However, they may be of importance in medicolegal situations, such as determination of paternity. An example is the MN group, which is a product of two genes (M and N). A person can therefore be MM, MN or NN, each genome coming from one parent. As with the other groups, analysis of the respective parties' genomes can only determine that the man is *not* the father. This method has been largely superceded by DNA profiling.

Complications of blood transfusions

Blood type incompatibility When the recipient of a blood transfusion has a significant plasma titre of α, β or anti-D antibodies, donor red cells expressing the respective antigen will rapidly agglutinate and haemolyse (**haemolytic transfusion reaction**). If the subsequent accumulation of bilirubin is sufficiently large, **haemolytic jaundice** develops. In severe cases renal failure may develop. Antibodies in the donor blood are rarely problematical, as they are diluted and removed in the recipient.

Transmission of infection as a result of bacteria, viruses and parasites. Most important are hepatitis, HIV, prions and in endemic areas parasites such as malaria.

Iron overload resulting from frequent transfusions and breakdown of red cells (*transfusion haemosiderosis*), for example in **thalassaemia** (see Chapter 6). Can cause damage to heart, liver, pancreas and glands. Treatment: iron chelators and vitamin C.

Fever resulting from an immune response to transfused leucocytes which release pyrogens. Relatively common but mild in patients who have previously been transfused, and in pregnancy.

Electrolyte changes and **suppression of haemostasis** following massive transfusions (e.g. major surgery) with stored blood (see below).

Blood storage

Blood is stored for transfusions at 4°C in the presence of an agent that chelates free Ca^{2+} to prevent clotting; for example, citrate, oxalate and ethylenediaminetetraacetic acid (EDTA; see Chapter 7). Even under these conditions the red cells deteriorate, although they last much longer in the presence of glucose, which provides a metabolic substrate. The cell membrane Na^+ pump works more slowly in the cold, with the result that Na^+ enters the cell, and K^+ leaves. This causes water to move into the cell so that it swells, and becomes more spherocytic. On prolonged storage the cells become fragile, and **haemolyse** (fragment) easily. Neither leucocytes nor platelets survive storage well, and disappear within a day of transfusion. Blood banks normally remove all the donor agglutinins (antibodies), although for small transfusions these would be sufficiently diluted to be of no threat. Great care is taken to screen potential donors for blood-borne diseases (e.g. hepatitis, HIV).

10 Membrane potential, ion channels and pumps

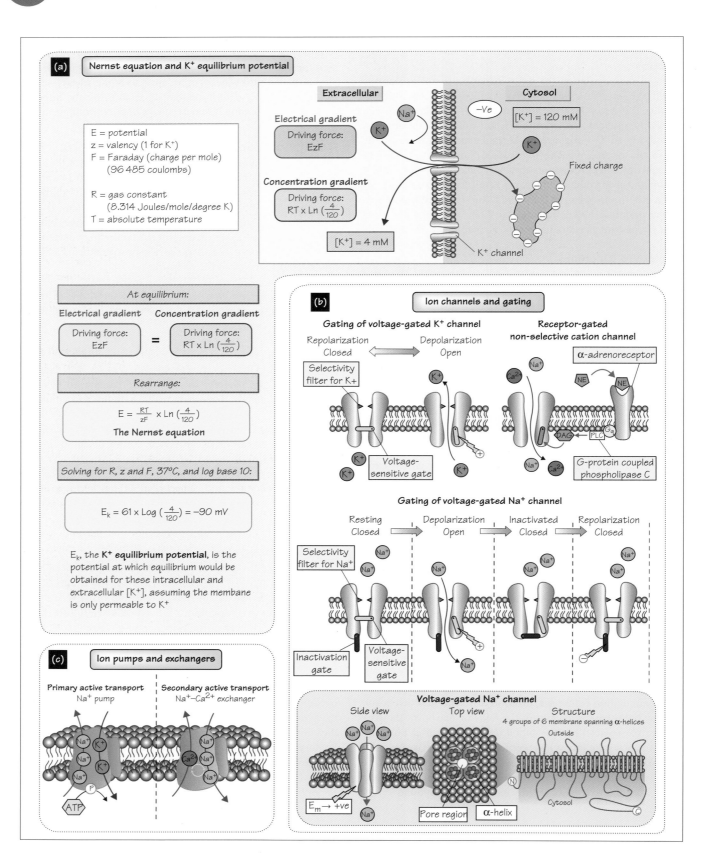

The Cardiovascular System at a Glance, Fourth Edition. Philip I. Aaronson, Jeremy P.T. Ward, and Michelle J. Connolly.

The cell membrane is a lipid bilayer with an intrinsically low permeability to charged ions. However, a variety of structures span the membrane through which ions can enter or leave the cell. These include **ion channels** through which ions passively diffuse and **ion pumps** which actively transport ions across the membrane. Pumps regulate ionic gradients, and channels determine membrane potential and underlie action potentials.

Resting membrane potential (Figure 10a)

The resting membrane is more permeable to K^+ and Cl^- than other ions, and is therefore **semipermeable**. The cell contains negatively charged molecules (e.g. proteins) which cannot cross the membrane. This fixed negative charge attracts K^+ but repels Cl^-, leading to accumulation of K^+ within the cell and loss of Cl^-. However, the consequent increase in K^+ concentration gradient drives K^+ back out of the cell. An equilibrium is reached when the *electrical* forces exactly balance those due to *concentration* differences (**Gibbs–Donnan equilibrium**); the net force or **electrochemical gradient** for K^+ is then zero. The opposing effect of the concentration gradient means fewer K^+ ions move into the cell than are required by the fixed negative charges. The inside of the cell is therefore negatively charged compared to the outside (*charge separation*), and a potential develops across the membrane. Only a small charge separation (e.g. 1 in ~100 000 K^+ ions) is required to cause a potential of ~-100 mV. If the membrane was only permeable to K^+ and no other cations, the potential at equilibrium (**K^+ equilibrium potential**, E_K) would be defined by the K^+ concentration gradient, and calculated from the **Nernst equation**. As cardiac muscle intracellular $[K^+]$ is ~120 mmol/L and extracellular $[K^+]$ ~4 mmol/L $E_K = $ ~-90 mV (Figure 10a).

In real membranes K^+ permeability (P_K) at rest is indeed greater than for other ions, so the **resting membrane potential** (RMP) is close to E_K (~-85 mV). RMP does not equal E_K because there is some permeability to other ions; most notably Na^+ permeability (P_{Na}) is ~1% of P_K. The Na^+ concentration gradient is also opposite to that for K^+ (intracellular $[Na^+]$ ~10 mmol/L, extracellular ~140 mmol/L), because the **Na^+ pump** (see below) actively removes Na^+ from the cell. As a result, the theoretical equilibrium potential for Na^+ (E_{Na}) is ~$+65$ mV, far from the actual RMP. Both concentration and electrical gradients are therefore in the same direction, and this inward **electrochemical gradient** drives Na^+ into the cell. As P_{Na} at rest is relatively low, the amount of Na^+ leaking into the cell is small, but is still sufficient to cause an inward current that slightly depolarizes the membrane. RMP is thus less negative than E_K. RMP can be calculated using the **Goldman equation**, a derivation of the Nernst equation taking into account other ions and their permeabilities.

A consequence of the above is that if P_{Na} was increased to more than P_K, then the membrane potential would shift towards E_{Na}. This is exactly what happens during an action potential, when Na^+ channels open so that P_{Na} becomes 10-fold greater than P_K, and the membrane depolarizes (see Chapter 11). An equivalent situation arises for Ca^{2+}, as intracellular $[Ca^{2+}]$ is ~100 nmol/L at rest, much smaller than the extracellular $[Ca^{2+}]$ of ~1 mmol/L.

Ion channels and gating (Figure 10b)

Channels differ in ion selectivity and activation mechanisms. They are either **open** or **closed**; transition between these states is called **gating**. When channels open ions move passively down their electrochemical gradient. As ions are charged, this causes an electrical current (***ionic current***); positive ions entering the cell cause **inward currents** and depolarization. Phosphorylation of channel proteins – by cAMP for example – can modify function, for example Ca^{2+} channels (see Chapter 11). There are several types of gating; two are described.

Voltage-gated channels (VGCs) are regulated by membrane potential. Some (e.g. certain K^+ channels) simply switch between **open** and **shut** states according to the potential across them (Figure 10b). Others, such as the **fast inward Na^+ channel** responsible for the upstroke of the action potential in nerves, skeletal and cardiac muscle (Figure 10b; see Chapter 11), have three states: open, shut and **inactive**. When a cell depolarizes sufficiently to activate these Na^+ channels (i.e. reaches their **threshold** potential), they open and the cell depolarizes towards E_{Na}. After a short period (<ms) the channels spontaneously **inactivate**, as though another gate had closed. Inactivated channels can only be reactivated once the membrane potential becomes negative again. This is essential for generation of action potentials (see Chapter 11).

Receptor-gated channels (RGCs; important in smooth muscle, see Chapter 15) are commonly **non-selective cation channels** (NSCCs; permeable to Na^+ and Ca^{2+}). They open when a hormone or neurotransmitter (e.g. noradrenaline) binds to a receptor and initiates production of a second messenger, such as **diacylglycerol** (DAG, Figure 10b).

Ion pumps and exchangers (Figure 10c)

Ion pumps use energy to transfer ions against their electrochemical gradient. **Primary active transport** consumes ATP for energy, the prime example being the **Na^+ pump** (Na^+–K^+-ATPase), which pumps three Na^+ out of the cell in exchange for two K^+. Another is the Ca^{2+}-ATPase that pumps Ca^{2+} into intracellular stores (see Chapters 12 and 15). **Secondary active transport** uses the Na^+ electrochemical gradient generated by the Na^+ pump to drive the transfer of other ions or molecules across the membrane. An example is the **Na^+–Ca^{2+} exchanger**, which exchanges three Na^+ ions for a Ca^{2+} ion (see Chapters 11 and 12). Na^+ pump inhibitors (e.g. **digoxin**) reduce the Na^+ gradient, and thus indirectly inhibit secondary transport. Pumps are regulated by ion concentrations, and modulated by second messengers.

Ion pumps and membrane potential

The Na^+ pump and Na^+–Ca^{2+} exchanger are **electrogenic** as unequal amounts of charge are transported, and thus a small ionic current is generated. They can therefore both affect, and be affected by, membrane potential. An example is Na^+–Ca^{2+} exchange during the cardiac muscle action potential (see Chapters 11 and 12).

11 Electrophysiology of cardiac muscle and origin of the heart beat

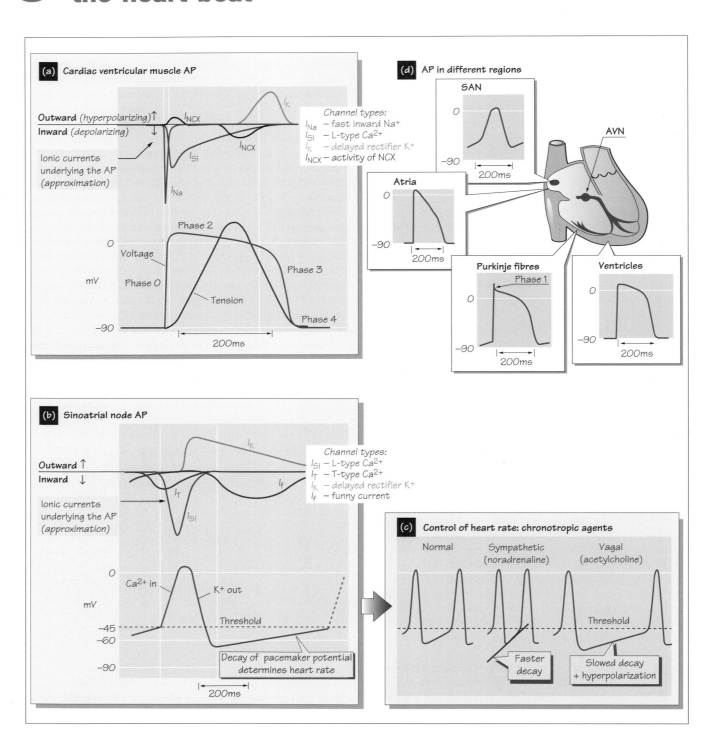

The Cardiovascular System at a Glance, Fourth Edition. Philip I. Aaronson, Jeremy P.T. Ward, and Michelle J. Connolly.
© 2013 John Wiley & Sons, Ltd. Published 2013 by John Wiley & Sons, Ltd.

An action potential (AP) is the transient depolarization of a cell as a result of activity of ion channels. The cardiac AP is considerably longer than those of nerve or skeletal muscle (~300 vs ~2 ms). This is due to a **plateau phase** in cardiac muscle, lasting for 200–300 ms.

Ventricular muscle action potential
(Figure 11a)
Initiation of the action potential
At rest, the ventricular cell membrane is most permeable to K^+ and the **resting membrane potential** (RMP) is therefore close to the K^+ equilibrium potential (E_K), ~–90 mV (see Chapter 10). An AP is initiated when the membrane is depolarized to the **threshold potential** (~–65 mV). This occurs due to transmission of a depolarizing current from an adjacent activated cell through **gap junctions** (see Chapter 2). At threshold, sufficient **voltage-gated Na^+ channels** are activated to initiate a self-regenerating process – the inward current caused by entry of Na^+ (I_{Na}) through these channels causes further depolarization, which activates more Na^+ channels, and so on. The outcome is a very large and fast I_{Na}, and therefore a very rapid AP upstroke (phase 0; ~500 V/s).

Activation of Na^+ channels during phase 0 means that the Na^+ permeability is now much greater than that for K^+, and so the membrane potential moves towards the Na^+ equilibrium potential (E_{Na}, ~+65 mV) (see Chapter 10). It does not reach E_{Na} because the Na^+ channels rapidly **inactivate** as the potential nears +40 mV (see Chapter 10); this, and activation of a transient outward K^+ current, can lead to a rapid decline in potential, leaving a spike (**phase 1**), best seen in Purkinje fibres (Figure 11d). The inactivated Na^+ channels cannot be **reactivated** until the potential returns to less than –60 mV, so another AP cannot be initiated until the cell repolarizes (**refractory period**). The refractory period therefore lasts as long as the plateau and contraction (Figure 11a), so unlike skeletal muscle, cardiac muscle cannot be tetanized.

The plateau (phase 2)
By the end of the upstroke all Na^+ channels are inactivated, and in skeletal muscle the cell would now repolarize. In cardiac muscle, however, the potential remains close to 0 mV for ~250 ms. This **plateau phase** is due to opening of **voltage-gated (L-type) Ca^{2+} channels**, which activate relatively slowly when the membrane potential becomes more positive than ~–35 mV. The resultant Ca^{2+} current (slow inward or I_{SI}) is sufficient to slow repolarization until the potential falls to ~–20 mV. The length of the plateau is related to slow **inactivation** of Ca^{2+} channels and the additional Na^+ inward current provided by the Na^+–Ca^{2+} exchanger (see below). Ca^{2+} entry during the plateau is vital for cardiac muscle contraction (see Chapter 12).

Repolarization (phase 3)
By the end of the plateau the membrane potential is sufficiently negative to activate *delayed rectifier* K^+ channels, and the associated outward K^+ current (I_K) therefore promotes rapid repolarization. As the membrane potential returns to resting levels (**phase 4**), I_K slowly inactivates again. Factors that influence I_K will affect the rate of repolarization, and hence the AP length (see Chapter 51), and mutations in the underlying channels cause long QT syndrome (see Chapter 55).

Role of Na^+–Ca^{2+} exchange
The Na^+–Ca^{2+} exchanger (NCX) exchanges three Na^+ for one Ca^{2+}, and is thus electrogenic (see Chapter 10). In the early plateau, when membrane potential is most positive, the NCX may reverse and contribute to inward current and movement of Ca^{2+}. As the plateau decays and becomes more negative NCX returns to its usual function of expelling Ca^{2+} from the cell in exchange for Na^+, which is potentiated by the high cytosolic [Ca^{2+}]. This influx of Na^+ ions causes an inward current (I_{NCX}) that slows repolarization and lengthens the plateau.

Sinoatrial node
The **sinoatrial node** (SAN) is the origin of the heart beat, and its AP differs from that of the ventricle (Figure 11b). The resting potential (phase 4) exhibits a slow depolarization, and the upstroke (phase 0) is much slower. The latter is because there are no functional Na^+ channels, and the upstroke is due instead to activation of slow L-type Ca^{2+} channels. The slow upstroke leads to slower conduction between cells (see Chapter 13). This is of particular importance in the **atrioventricular node** (AVN), which has a similar AP to the SAN.

The SAN resting potential slowly depolarizes from ~–60 mV to a threshold of ~–40 mV, at which point L-type channels activate and an AP is initiated; the threshold is more positive because of substitution of L-type for Na^+ channels. The rate of decay determines how long it takes for threshold to be reached, and therefore the heart rate. The resting potential is therefore commonly called the **pacemaker potential**. As for ventricular cells, repolarization of the AP in SAN involves activation of I_K, which then slowly inactivates. In addition, there are two inward currents, I_b and I_f ('*funny*'), mostly due to inward movement of Na^+. I_b is stable, and present in other cardiac cells, but I_f is specific to nodal cells, and activated at the end of repolarization by negative potentials (Figure 11b). The combination of inward current from I_f plus I_b and decay in I_K causes the slow depolarization of the pacemaker potential. As this approaches threshold, another type of voltage-gated Ca^{2+} channel (transient, T-type) is activated, which contributes to the depolarization and the early part of the upstroke.

Factors influencing I_K, I_b, or I_f thus alter the slope of the pacemaker and so heart rate, and are called **chronotropic agents**. The sympathetic neurotransmitter noradrenaline increases heart rate by increasing the size of I_f. It also reduces AP length by increasing the rate of Ca^{2+} entry and hence the slope of the upstroke. The parasympathetic transmitter acetylcholine reduces the slope of the pacemaker potential and causes a small hyperpolarization, both of which increase the time required to reach threshold and reduce heart rate (Figure 11c).

Other regions of the heart (Figure 11d)
Atrial muscle has a similar AP to ventricular muscle, although the shape is more triangular. **Purkinje fibres** in the conduction system have a prominent phase 1, reflecting a greater I_{Na} (due to their large size); the latter causes a more rapid upstroke, and faster conduction. APs in the AVN are similar to those of the SAN, although the rate of decay of the resting potential is slower. The resting potential of the bundle of His and Purkinje system may also exhibit an even slower rate of decay (due to decay of I_K). All of these could therefore act as pacemakers, but the SAN is normally faster and predominates. This is called **dominance** or **overdrive suppression**.

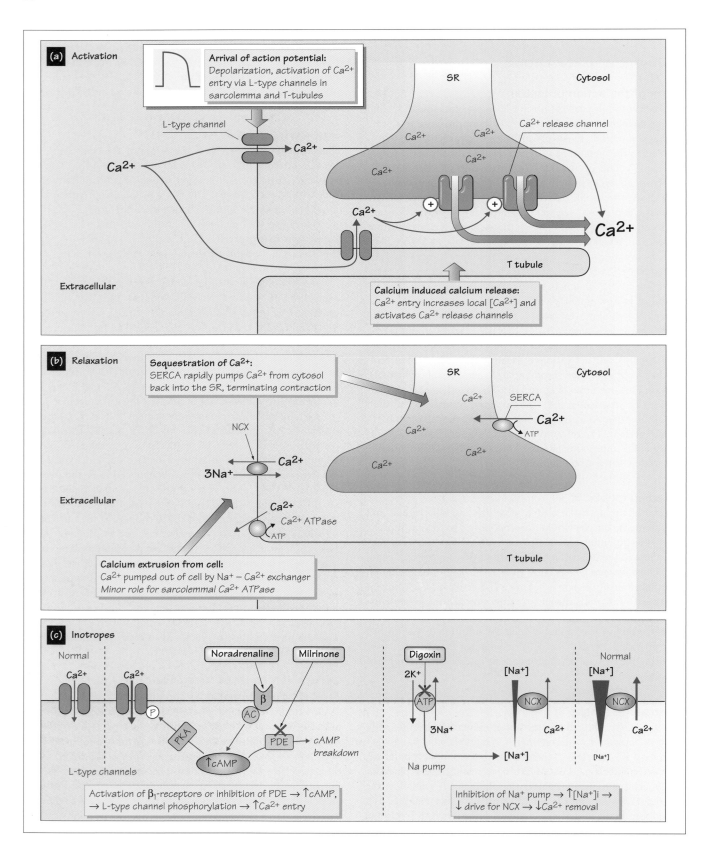

The Cardiovascular System at a Glance, Fourth Edition. Philip I. Aaronson, Jeremy P.T. Ward, and Michelle J. Connolly.

Cardiac muscle contracts when cytosolic $[Ca^{2+}]$ rises above about 100 nmol/L. This rise in $[Ca^{2+}]$ couples the action potential (AP) to contraction, and the mechanisms involved are referred to as **excitation–contraction coupling**. The relationship between cardiac muscle force and stretch is discussed in Chapter 17. The ability of cardiac muscle to generate force *for any given fibre length* is described as its **contractility**. This depends on cytosolic $[Ca^{2+}]$, and to a lesser extent on factors that affect Ca^{2+} sensitivity of the contractile apparatus. The contractility of cardiac muscle is primarily dependent on the way that the cell handles Ca^{2+}.

Initiation of contraction

During the **plateau phase** of the AP, Ca^{2+} enters the cell through L-**type voltage-gated Ca^{2+} channels** (Figure 12). L-type channels are specifically blocked by **dihydropyridines** (e.g. **nifedipine**) and *verapamil*. However, the amount of Ca^{2+} that enters the cell is less than 20% of that required for the observed rise in cytosolic $[Ca^{2+}]$ ($[Ca^{2+}]_i$). The rest is released from the **sarcoplasmic reticulum** (SR), where Ca^{2+} is stored in high concentrations associated with **calsequestrin**. APs travels down the **T tubules** which are close to, but do not touch, the **terminal cisternae** of the SR (Figure 12a). During the first 1–2 ms of the plateau Ca^{2+} enters and causes a rise in $[Ca^{2+}]$ in the gap between the T tubule sarcolemma and SR. This rise in $[Ca^{2+}]$ activates Ca^{2+}-sensitive **Ca^{2+} release channels** in the SR, through which stored Ca^{2+} floods into the cytoplasm. This is called **calcium-induced calcium release (CICR)** (Figure 12a). The amount of Ca^{2+} released depends both on the content of the SR and size of the activating Ca^{2+} entry, and modulation of the latter is the major way by which cardiac function is regulated (see Regulation of contractility below). Ca^{2+} release and entry combine to cause a rapid increase in $[Ca^{2+}]_i$, which initiates contraction. Peak $[Ca^{2+}]_i$ normally rises to ~2 μmol/L, although maximum contraction occurs when $[Ca^{2+}]_i$ rises above 10 μmol/L.

Generation of tension

The arrangement of **actin** and **myosin** filaments is discussed in Chapter 2. Force is generated when myosin heads protruding from thick filaments bind to actin thin filaments to form **crossbridges**, and drag the actin past in a ratchet fashion, using ATP bound to myosin as an energy source. This is the **sliding filament** or **crossbridge mechanism** of muscle contraction. In cardiac muscle $[Ca^{2+}]_i$ controls crossbridge formation via the regulatory proteins **tropomyosin** and **troponin**. Tropomyosin is a coiled strand which, at rest, lies in the cleft between the two actin chains that form the thin filament helix, and covers the myosin binding sites. Myosin therefore cannot bind, and there is no tension. Troponin is a complex of three globular proteins (**troponin C, I and T**), bound to tropomyosin by **troponin T** at intervals of 40 nm. When $[Ca^{2+}]_i$ rises above 100 nmol/L, Ca^{2+} binds to **troponin C** causing a conformational change which allows tropomyosin to shift out of the actin cleft. Myosin binding sites are uncovered, myosin crossbridges form and tension develops. Tension is related to the number of active crossbridges, and will increase until all troponin C is bound to Ca^{2+} ($[Ca^{2+}]_i > 10$ μmol/L).

Relaxation mechanisms

When $[Ca^{2+}]_i$ rises above resting levels (~100 nmol/L), ATP-dependent Ca^{2+} pumps in the SR (sarcoendoplasmic reticulum Ca^{2+}-ATPase; **SERCA**) are activated, and start to pump (**sequester**) Ca^{2+} from the cytosol back into the SR (Figure 12b). As the AP repolarizes and L-type Ca^{2+} channels inactivate, this mechanism reduces $[Ca^{2+}]_i$ towards resting levels, so Ca^{2+} dissociates from troponin C and the muscle relaxes. However, the Ca^{2+} originally entering the cell must now be expelled. Ca^{2+} is transported out of the cell by the membrane **Na$^+$–Ca^{2+} exchanger** (NCX) (see Chapters 10 and 11). This uses the inward Na$^+$ electrochemical gradient as an energy source to pump Ca^{2+} out, and three Na$^+$ enter the cell for each Ca^{2+} removed (Figure 12b). Sarcolemmal Ca^{2+}-ATPase pumps are present but less important. At the end of the AP about 80% of the Ca^{2+} will have been resequestered into the SR, and most of the rest ejected from the cell. The remainder is slowly pumped out between beats.

Regulation of contractility

Inotropic agents alter the contractility of cardiac muscle; a positive inotrope increases contractility, while a negative decreases it. Most inotropes act by modulating cell Ca^{2+} handling, although some may alter Ca^{2+} binding to troponin C. A high plasma $[Ca^{2+}]$ increases contractility by increasing Ca^{2+} entry during the AP.

Noradrenaline from sympathetic nerve endings, and to a lesser extent circulating **adrenaline**, are the most important physiological inotropic agents. They also increase heart rate (positive **chronotropes**; see Chapter 11). Noradrenaline binds to β$_1$-adrenoceptors on the sarcolemma and activates adenylate cyclase (AC), causing production of the second messenger cAMP. This activates protein kinase A (PKA), which phosphorylates L-type Ca^{2+} channels so that they allow more Ca^{2+} to enter during the AP (Figure 12c; see Chapter 11). The elevation of $[Ca^{2+}]_i$ is thus potentiated and more force develops. Any agent that increases cAMP will act as a positive inotrope, for example milrinone, an inhibitor of the phosphodiesterase that breaks down cAMP. Noradrenaline (and cAMP) also increase the rate of Ca^{2+} reuptake into the SR, mediated by PKA and phosphorylation of **phospholamban**, a SERCA regulatory protein. While not affecting contractility, this assists removal of the additional Ca^{2+} and shortens contraction, which is useful for high heart rates.

The classic positive inotropic drug is **digoxin**, a **cardiac glycoside**. Digoxin inhibits the **Na$^+$ pump** (Na$^+$-K$^+$ ATPase) which removes [Na$^+$] from cells. Intracellular [Na$^+$] therefore increases, so reducing the Na$^+$ gradient that drives NCX (see Chapter 11). Consequently, less Ca^{2+} is removed from the cell by the NCX (Figure 12c) and peak $[Ca^{2+}]_i$ and force increase.

Overstimulation by positive inotropes can lead to **Ca^{2+} overload**, and damage due to excessive uptake of Ca^{2+} by the SR and mitochondria. This can contribute to the progressive decline in myocardial function in **chronic heart failure** (see Chapter 46), when sympathetic stimulation is high.

Acidosis is *negatively* inotropic, largely by interfering with the actions of Ca^{2+}. This is important in **myocardial ischaemia** and **heart failure**, where poor perfusion can lead to **lactic acidosis** and so depress cardiac function.

Influence of heart rate

When heart rate increases there is a proportional rise in cardiac muscle force. This phenomenon is known as the **staircase**, **Treppe** or **Bowditch** effect. It can be attributed both to an increase in cytosolic [Na$^+$] due to the greater frequency of APs, with a consequent inhibition of NCX (see above), and to a decreased diastolic interval, which limits the time between beats for Ca^{2+} to be extruded from the cell.

13 Electrical conduction system in the heart

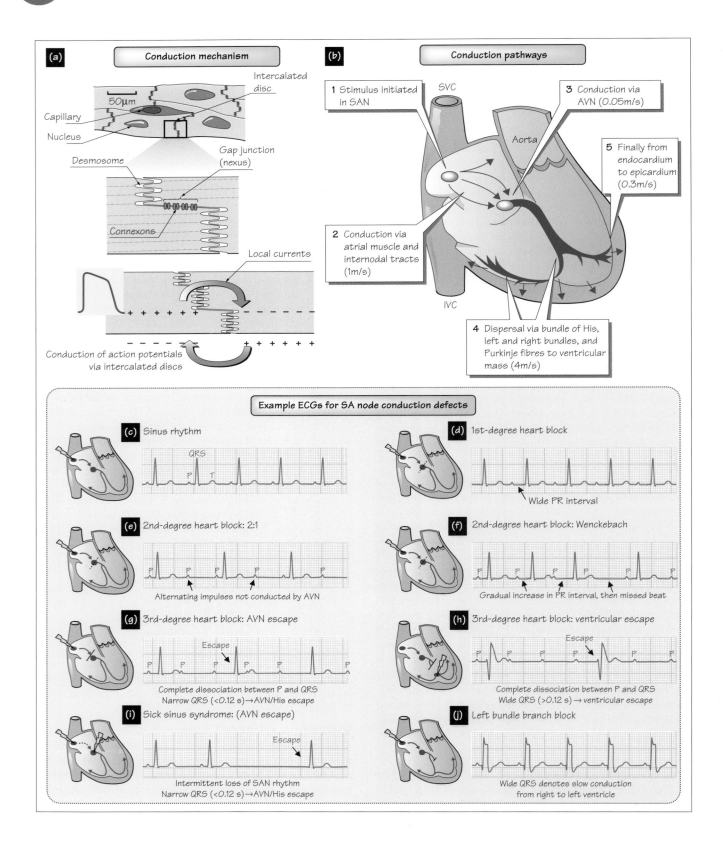

(a) Conduction mechanism

- Intercalated disc
- 50μm
- Capillary
- Nucleus
- Desmosome
- Gap junction (nexus)
- Connexons
- Local currents
- Conduction of action potentials via intercalated discs

(b) Conduction pathways

- SVC
- Aorta
- IVC
- 1 Stimulus initiated in SAN
- 2 Conduction via atrial muscle and internodal tracts (1m/s)
- 3 Conduction via AVN (0.05m/s)
- 4 Dispersal via bundle of His, left and right bundles, and Purkinje fibres to ventricular mass (4m/s)
- 5 Finally from endocardium to epicardium (0.3m/s)

Example ECGs for SA node conduction defects

(c) Sinus rhythm
QRS
P T

(d) 1st-degree heart block
Wide PR interval

(e) 2nd-degree heart block: 2:1
P P P P P
Alternating impulses not conducted by AVN

(f) 2nd-degree heart block: Wenckebach
P P P P P
Gradual increase in PR interval, then missed beat

(g) 3rd-degree heart block: AVN escape
Escape
P P P P P P
Complete dissociation between P and QRS
Narrow QRS (<0.12 s)→AVN/His escape

(h) 3rd-degree heart block: ventricular escape
Escape
P P P P P P
Complete dissociation between P and QRS
Wide QRS (>0.12 s) → ventricular escape

(i) Sick sinus syndrome: (AVN escape)
Escape
Intermittent loss of SAN rhythm
Narrow QRS (<0.12 s)→AVN/His escape

(j) Left bundle branch block
Wide QRS denotes slow conduction from right to left ventricle

The Cardiovascular System at a Glance, Fourth Edition. Philip I. Aaronson, Jeremy P.T. Ward, and Michelle J. Connolly.

Electrical conduction in cardiac muscle
(Figure 13a)

Cardiac muscle cells are connected via **intercalated discs** (see Chapter 2). These incorporate regions where the membranes of adjacent cells are very close, called **gap junctions.** Gap junctions consist of proteins known as **connexons**, which form low-resistance junctions between cells. They allow the transfer of small ions and thus electrical current. As all cells are therefore electrically connected, cardiac muscle is said to be a **functional** (or electrical) **syncytium.** If an action potential (AP) is initiated in one cell, local currents via gap junctions will cause adjacent cells to depolarize, initiating their own AP. A wave of depolarization will therefore be conducted from cell to cell throughout the myocardium. The rate of conduction is partly dependent on gap junction resistance and the *size of the depolarizing current.* This is related to the **upstroke velocity of the AP** (phase 0). Drugs that slow phase 0 therefore slow conduction (e.g. lidocaine, class I antiarrhythmics). Pathological conditions such as ischaemia may increase gap junction resistance, and slow or abolish conduction. Retrograde conduction does not normally occur because the original cell is refractory (see Chapter 11). Transfer of the pacemaker signal from the sinoatrial node (SAN) and synchronous contraction of the ventricles is facilitated by **conduction pathways** formed from modified muscle cells.

Conduction pathways in the heart
(Figure 13b)
Sinoatrial node

The heart beat is normally initiated in the **SAN**, located at the junction of the superior vena cava and right atrium. The SAN is a ~2-mm-wide group of small elongated muscle cells that extends for ~2 cm down the sulcus terminalis. It has a rich capillary supply and sympathetic and parasympathetic (right vagal) nerve endings. The SAN generates an AP about once a second (sinus rhythm, Figure 13c; see Chapter 11).

Atrial conduction

The impulse spreads from the SAN across the atria at ~1 m/s. Conduction to the **atrioventricular node** (AVN) is facilitated by larger cells in the three **internodal tracts** of Bachmann (anterior), Wenckebach (middle) and Thorel (posterior).

The atrioventricular node

The atria and ventricles are separated by the non-conducting **annulus fibrosus.** The AVN marks the upper region of the only conducting route through this band. It is similar in structure to the SAN, situated near the interatrial septum and mouth of the coronary sinus, and innervated by sympathetic and left vagal nerves. The complex arrangement of small cells and slow AP upstroke (see Chapter 11) result in a very slow conduction velocity (~0.05 m/s). This provides a functionally significant delay of ~0.1 s between contraction of the atria and ventricles, reflected by the **PR interval** of the electrocardiogram (**ECG;** see Chapter 14). Sympathetic stimulation increases conduction velocity and reduces the delay, whereas vagal stimulation slows conduction and increases the delay.

Bundle of His and Purkinje system

The **bundle of His** transfers the impulse from the AVN to the top of the interventricular septum. Close to the attachment of the tricuspid septal cusp it branches to form the **left** and **right bundle branches**. The left bundle divides into the posterior and anterior fascicles. The bundles travel under the endocardium down the walls of the septum, and at the base divide into the multiple fibres of the **Purkinje system.** This distributes the impulse over the inner walls of the ventricles. Cells in the bundle of His and Purkinje system have large diameters (~40 μm) and rapid AP upstroke, and consequently fast conduction (~4 m/s). The impulse spreads from the Purkinje cells through the endocardium towards the epicardium at 0.3–1 m/s, thereby initiating contraction.

Abnormalities of impulse generation or conduction (see also Chapters 48–50)

Sinus tachycardia (100–200 beats/min) is normal in exercise or excitement, but also occurs when pathological stimuli (e.g. phaeochromocytoma, heart failure, thyrotoxicosis) elevate sympathetic tone and accelerate SAN firing. Sinus tachycardia generally starts and stops gradually. Treatment, if required, involves removing the underlying cause. The ECG is otherwise normal. Conversely, **sick sinus syndrome**, generally caused by SAN fibrosis, causes slowed impulse generation and **bradycardia** (slow heart rate), or a sustained or intermittent failure of the impulse to reach the AVN, termed **sinoatrial block** (Figure 13i). Because other parts of the conduction system also exhibit pacemaking activity (see Chapter 11), sick sinus syndrome can result in the emergence of **escape** beats or rhythms in which impulses arising elsewhere (usually the AVN) can activate ventricular depolarization. Sick sinus syndrome can be treated by implantation of a pacemaker.

Heart block Abnormally slow conduction in the AVN can result in incomplete (**first-degree**) heart block (*AV block*; Figure 13d), where the delay is greater than normal, resulting in an extended PR interval. **Second-degree** heart block occurs when only a fraction of impulses from the atria are conducted; for example, ventricular contraction is only initiated every second or third atrial contraction (**2:1 or 3:1 block**; Mobitz II; Figure 13e). **Wenckebach block** (Mobitz I) is another type of second-degree block, in which the PR interval progressively lengthens until there is no transmission from atria to ventricles and a QRS complex is missed; the cycle then begins again (Figure 13f). Patients with first or second-degree block are often asymptomatic. Complete (**third-degree**) heart block occurs when conduction between atria and ventricles is abolished (Figure 13g,h). This can result from ischaemic damage to nodal tissue or the bundle of His. In the absence of a signal from the SAN, the AVN and bundle of His can generate a heart rate of ~40 beats/min (see Chapter 11). Some ventricular cells spontaneously generate APs, but at a rate less than 20/min.

Bundle branch block When one branch of the bundle of His does not conduct (*left or right bundle branch block*), the part of the ventricle that it serves will be stimulated by conduction through the myocardium from unaffected areas. As this form of conduction is slower, activation is delayed and the QRS complex broadened, often with a more prominent Q wave (Figure 13j).

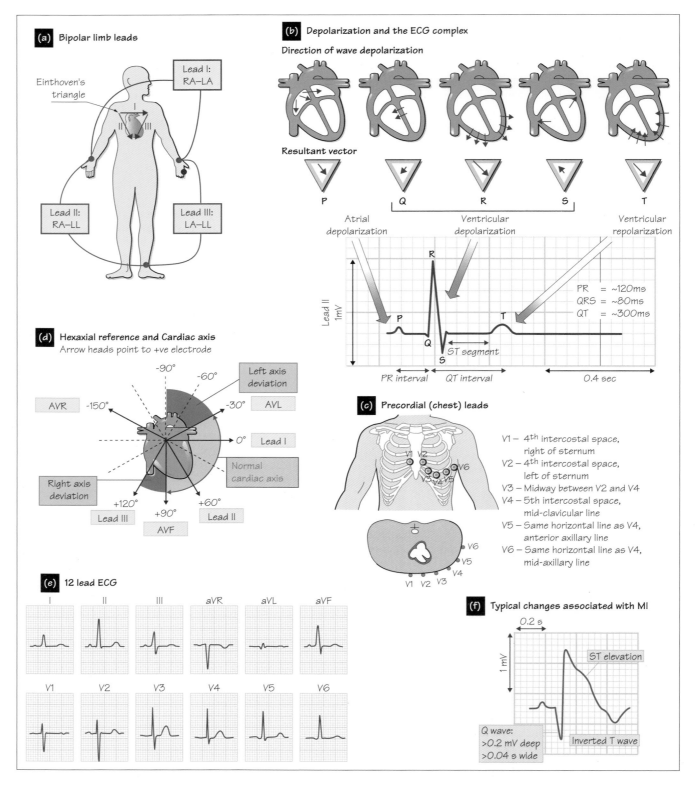

(a) Bipolar limb leads

Einthoven's triangle

Lead I: RA–LA

Lead II: RA–LL

Lead III: LA–LL

(b) Depolarization and the ECG complex

Direction of wave depolarization

Resultant vector

P   Q   R   S   T

Atrial depolarization   Ventricular depolarization   Ventricular repolarization

Lead II 1mV

R

P   T

Q

S   ST segment

PR interval   QT interval   0.4 sec

PR = ~120ms
QRS = ~80ms
QT = ~300ms

(d) Hexaxial reference and Cardiac axis

Arrow heads point to +ve electrode

-90°
-60°
-30°
AVR -150°
AVL
0° Lead I
Left axis deviation
Normal cardiac axis
Right axis deviation
+120° +60°
+90°
Lead III   Lead II
AVF

(c) Precordial (chest) leads

V1 V2
V6
V3 V4 V5

V1 – 4th intercostal space, right of sternum
V2 – 4th intercostal space, left of sternum
V3 – Midway between V2 and V4
V4 – 5th intercostal space, mid-clavicular line
V5 – Same horizontal line as V4, anterior axillary line
V6 – Same horizontal line as V4, mid-axillary line

V6
V5
V4
V1 V2 V3

(e) 12 lead ECG

I   II   III   aVR   aVL   aVF

V1   V2   V3   V4   V5   V6

(f) Typical changes associated with MI

0.2 s

1 mV

ST elevation

Q wave:
>0.2 mV deep
>0.04 s wide

Inverted T wave

The **electrocardiogram** (ECG) is the surface recording of electrical activity of the heart as the cardiac muscle depolarizes and repolarizes (see Chapters 11 and 13). The recorded voltage (1–2 mV) is much smaller than that of the action potential, and reflects the *vector sum* of currents between depolarized and resting cells, thus providing both **amplitude** and **directional** information. Identifica-

The Cardiovascular System at a Glance, Fourth Edition. Philip I. Aaronson, Jeremy P.T. Ward, and Michelle J. Connolly.

tion of intermittent events such as paroxysmal arrhythmias may require ambulatory ECG recording over 24 hours (**Holter** test), or an **exercise tolerance test** where workload is progressively increased to elicit events related to coronary artery disease for example.

Recording the ECG

The ECG is based around the concept of an equilateral triangle (**Einthoven's triangle**; Figure 14a). The points of the triangle are approximated by placing electrodes on the right arm (RA), left arm (LA) and left leg (LL). The right leg is commonly used as an earth to minimize interference. The voltage between any two electrodes will depend on the amplitude of the current, which is related to muscle mass, and the mean direction of current; it is thus a **vector quantity** (Figure 14b). The greatest voltage and thus deflection is therefore seen when the wave of depolarization is directly towards or away from the respective electrodes. By convention, the ECG is connected such that a wave of depolarization towards the positive electrode causes an upward deflection, and the paper speed of the recorder is normally 25 or 50 mm/s.

The various combinations of electrodes are called **leads** (not to be confused with the cables connecting the electrodes). The three **bipolar limb leads** each approximate the potential difference (PD) between two corners of Einthoven's triangle, and are essentially looking at electrical activity in the heart from three different directions, separated by 60°. **Lead I** measures the PD between RA (positive electrode) and LA (negative electrode); **lead II**, RA (negative) and LL (positive); and **lead III**, LA (negative) and LL (positive).

The **unipolar leads** use a single sensing electrode, and measure the PD between this and an **indifferent electrode** representing the average potential of the whole body (i.e. zero). Practically, this is obtained by connecting RA, LA and LL together, which approximates the centre of Einthoven's triangle (i.e. the heart). The six **precordial** (chest) leads use a separate *sensing* (positive) electrode placed on the chest so as to accentuate activity in particular regions of the heart (Figure 14c): V1 and V2, right ventricle; V3 and V4, interventricular septum; V5 and V6, left ventricle. However, the **augmented** limb leads use one limb connection as the sensing electrode (aVR, RA; aVL, LA; aVF, LL), with the remaining two connected together as the indifferent electrode. As they therefore measure from each corner of Einthoven's triangle towards the centre, they 'see' the heart at angles rotated by 30° compared with the bipolar leads. The six limb leads therefore give a view of the electrical activity of the heart every 30° (**hexaxial reference system**; Figure 14d). Lead II and AVR normally shows the tallest QRS, as they lie closest to the mean direction of ventricular depolarization; as the ventricles have the greatest muscle mass, they generate the largest current. Together, the limb and precordial leads provide the standard **12 lead ECG** (Figure 14e).

General features of the ECG (Figure 14b)

The **P wave** (≤0.12 s duration) is a small deflection due to depolarization of the atria (atrial systole). The **QRS complex** is normally <0.08 s in duration and reflects ventricular depolarization; it is largest because of the large ventricular mass. The relative size of the individual components varies between leads. In lead II the **Q wave** is a small downward deflection, reflecting left to right depolarization of the interventricular septum. The **R wave** is a strong upwards deflection, reflecting depolarization of the main ventricular mass. The **S wave** is a small downward deflection in lead II,

and reflects depolarization of the last part of the ventricle close to the base of the heart. The **T wave** reflects ventricular repolarization, and is normally in the same direction as the R wave (e.g. upwards deflection in lead II). This is because although it is opposite in polarity, its *direction* is the opposite of that for depolarization (Figure 14b), as the length of action potential in the epicardium is shorter than that in the endocardium, so although the epicardium depolarizes last it repolarizes first. The reversal in direction therefore cancels out the reversal in polarity. Note that atrial repolarization is too small and diffuse to be seen, and the conducting system (see Chapter 13) has too small a mass to generate any significant voltage.

The **PR interval** represents the delay between atrial and ventricular depolarization, mostly in the atrioventricular node (AVN), and is measured from the start of P to the start of QRS. Normal duration is 0.12–0.20 s. The **ST segment** (~0.25 s) is normally **isoelectric** (i.e. at zero potential), because all ventricular muscle is depolarized and so there can be no current flow between cells. The **QT interval**, from the start of QRS to the end of T, represents the duration of ventricular activation. It is strongly dependent on heart rate and is generally corrected by the **Bazett formula** ($QT_C = QT$/square root of R–R interval). QT_C is normally <0.44 s, slightly longer in females.

Basic interpretation of the ECG (Figure 14e)

Rate and rhythm Heart rate in beats/min is 1/RR interval × 60. At a paper speed of 25 mm/s one large square = 0.2 s, one small square = 0.04 s. A heart rate above 100 beats/min is **tachycardia**, and below 60 beats/min **bradycardia**. A regular rhythm with a constant normal PR interval is **sinus rhythm**. A prolonged PR interval or disassociation of P and QRS waves suggests impaired conduction in the AVN or bundle of His (see Chapter 13).

QRS A broad and negative **Q wave** (sometimes normal in AVR and V1) or broad and misshapen QRS can be caused by a number of defects, including bundle branch block (see Chapter 13) or a ventricular origin of the heart beat (e.g. ectopic beats). A slowly developing Q wave may indicate a full wall-thickness **myocardial infarction** (MI; Figure 14f; see Chapter 45).

Cardiac axis The direction of maximum ECG amplitude (mean vector), and thus of the sum of currents generated by the ventricles. It is calculated from the relative size of the QRS for each limb lead, and ranges from +90° to −30° (Figure 14d). It depends on the orientation of the heart and so varies during breathing. **Left axis deviation** (−30° to −90°) may reflect left ventricular hypertrophy, and **right axis deviation** (+90° to +120°) right ventricular hypertrophy.

ST segment elevation Due to **injury currents** between damaged and undamaged cells, normally transient and indicative of recent MI (Figure 14f; see Chapter 45). Subendocardial MI may cause ST segment **depression**.

T wave inversion Often normal in lead III and V1, but in other leads may reflect MI and slowed conduction, such that repolarization of the epicardium occurs before repolarization of the endocardium. A **tall peaked T wave** can be caused by hyperkalaemia.

Prolonged QT_C Reflects delayed repolarisation, and can be caused by class IA and III antiarrhythmic drugs, heart failure and inherited long QT syndrome (see Chapters 46, 51 and 54).

15 Vascular smooth muscle excitation–contraction coupling

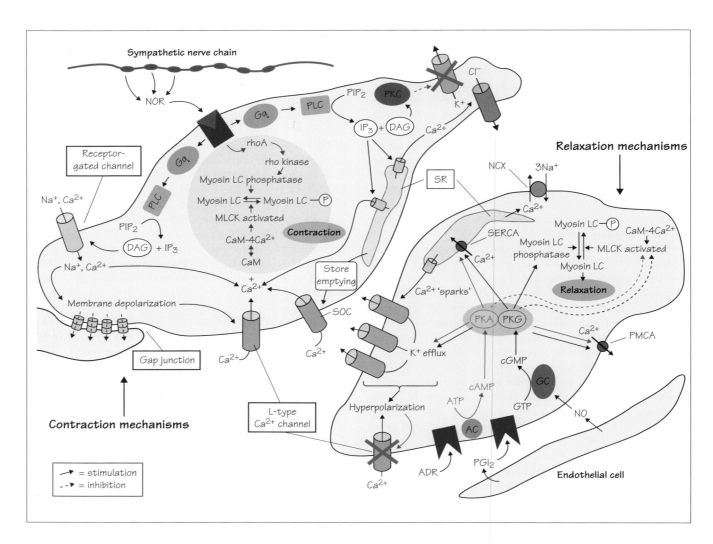

Vascular smooth muscle (VSM) contraction is, like that of cardiac muscle, controlled by the *intracellular Ca^{2+} concentration* $[Ca^{2+}]_i$. Unlike cardiac muscle cells, however, VSM cells lack troponin and utilize a *myosin-based system* to regulate contraction.

Regulation of contraction by Ca^{2+} and myosin phosphorylation (see shaded area in left cell of Figure 15)

Vasoconstricting stimuli initiate VSM cell contraction by increasing $[Ca^{2+}]_i$ from its basal level of ~100 nmol/L. Force development is proportional to the increase in $[Ca^{2+}]_i$, with maximal contraction occurring at ~1 µmol/L $[Ca^{2+}]_i$. The rise in $[Ca^{2+}]_i$ promotes its binding to the cytoplasmic regulatory protein **calmodulin (CaM)**. Once a calmodulin molecule has bound four Ca^{2+} ions, it can activate the enzyme **myosin light-chain kinase (MLCK)**. MLCK in turn phosphorylates two 20-kDa subunits (**'light chains'**) contained within the 'head' of each myosin molecule. Phosphorylated myosin

then forms crossbridges with actin, using ATP hydrolysis as an energy source to produce contraction. Actin–myosin interactions during crossbridge cycling are similar to those in cardiac myocytes (see Chapter 12).

The degree of myosin light-chain phosphorylation, which determines crossbridge turnover, is a balance between the activity of MLCK and a **myosin light-chain phosphatase** which dephosphorylates the light chains. Once $[Ca^{2+}]_i$ falls, MLCK activity diminishes and relaxation occurs as light-chain phosphorylation is returned to basal levels by the phosphatase.

VSM cells *in vivo* maintain a tonic level of partial contraction that varies with fluctuations in the vasoconstricting and vasodilating influences to which they are exposed. VSM cells avoid fatigue during prolonged contractions because their rate of ATP consumption is 300-fold lower than that of skeletal muscle fibres. This is possible because the crossbridge cycle is much slower than in striated muscles. The maximum crossbridge cycling rate of smooth

The Cardiovascular System at a Glance, Fourth Edition. Philip I. Aaronson, Jeremy P.T. Ward, and Michelle J. Connolly.

muscle during shortening is only about one-tenth of that in striated muscles, as a result of differences in the types of myosin present. In addition, once they have shortened, vascular cells can maintain contraction with an even lower expenditure of ATP because the myosin crossbridges remain attached to actin for a longer time, thus 'locking in' shortening.

Vasoconstricting mechanisms

The binding to receptors of **noradrenaline** and other important vasoconstrictors such as **endothelin, thromboxane A₂, angiotensin II** and **vasopressin** stimulates VSM contraction via common **G-protein-mediated** pathways (see left cell).

Effects of IP₃ and diacylglycerol

Binding of vasoconstrictors to receptors activates the G-protein **Gq**, which stimulates the enzyme **phospholipase C**. Phospholipase C splits the membrane phospholipid phosphatidylinositol 1,4-bisphosphate (PIP₂), generating the second messengers inositol 1,4,5-triphosphate (**IP₃**), and diacylglycerol (**DAG**). IP₃ binds to and opens Ca^{2+} channels on the membrane of the **sarcoplasmic reticulum** (SR). This allows Ca^{2+}, which is stored in high concentrations within the SR, to flood out into the cytoplasm and rapidly increase $[Ca^{2+}]_i$. DAG activates **protein kinase C** (PKC). This activates the protein **CPI-17**, which phosphorylates and inhibits myosin phosphatase, promoting contraction.

Ca²⁺ influx mechanisms

Vasoconstrictors also cause **membrane depolarization** via several mechanisms. First, the release of SR Ca^{2+}, which they initiate, opens Ca^{2+}-**activated chloride channels** in the plasma membrane. Second, vasoconstrictors may act via DAG and PKC to cause depolarization by *inhibiting* the activity of **K⁺ channels**. Third, vasoconstrictors induce both membrane depolarization and Ca^{2+} entry into VSM cells by opening **receptor-gated cation channels**, which allow the influx of both Na⁺ and Ca^{2+} ions. The identities of the proteins making up the Ca^{2+}-activated chloride and receptor-gated cation channels remained elusive for many years, but these channels have recently been proposed to be formed from **anoctamin** and **TRPC** (transient receptor potential canonical) proteins, respectively.

The membrane depolarization elicited by vasoconstrictors opens **L-type voltage-gated Ca²⁺ channels** (also termed Ca_V 1.2 channels) similar to those found in cardiac myocytes. With sufficient depolarization, some blood vessels may fire brief Ca^{2+} channel-mediated APs that cause transient contractions. More often, however, vasoconstrictors cause graded depolarizations, during which sufficient Ca^{2+} influx occurs to cause more sustained contractions. Vasoconstrictors further enhance Ca^{2+} influx through L-type channels by evoking channel phosphorylation. Furthermore, depletion of Ca^{2+} from the SR due to the action of IP₃ opens **store-operated Ca²⁺ (SOC) channels** in the cell membrane which admit both Na⁺ and Ca^{2+} into the cell. The identities of the proteins forming SOC channels remain in dispute.

As well as raising $[Ca^{2+}]_i$, vasoconstrictors also promote contraction by a process termed **Ca²⁺ sensitization**. Ca^{2+} sensitization is caused by the inhibition of myosin phosphatase. This increases myosin light-chain phosphorylation, and therefore force development, even with minimal increases in $[Ca^{2+}]_i$ and MLCK activity.

Although PKC has this effect (see above), phosphatase inhibition is primarily caused by **RhoA kinase**, an enzyme stimulated by the *ras* type G-protein **RhoA**, which is activated by vasoconstrictors by an as yet unknown mechanism.

The relative importance of the excitatory mechanisms listed above varies between different vasoconstrictors and vascular beds. In resistance arteries depolarization and Ca^{2+} influx through voltage-gated channels are probably most important.

Ca²⁺ removal and vasodilator mechanisms
(see right cell of Figure 15)

Several mechanisms serve to remove Ca^{2+} from the cytoplasm. These are continually active, allowing cells both to recover from stimulation and to maintain a low basal $[Ca^{2+}]_i$ in the face of the enormous electrochemical gradient tending to drive Ca^{2+} into cells even when they are not stimulated. The **smooth endoplasmic reticulum Ca²⁺-ATPase (SERCA)** pumps Ca^{2+} from the cytoplasm into the SR. This process is referred to as **Ca²⁺ sequestration**. An analogous **plasma membrane Ca²⁺-ATPase (PMCA)** pumps Ca^{2+} from the cytoplasm into the extracellular space (**Ca²⁺ extrusion**). Cells also extrude Ca^{2+} via a **Na⁺-Ca²⁺ exchanger (NCX)** located in the cell membrane, which is similar to that found in cardiac cells (see Chapter 12). The NCX may be localized to areas of the plasma membrane that are approached closely by the SR, allowing any Ca^{2+} leaking from the SR to be quickly ejected from the cell without causing tension development. Interestingly, when the intracellular Na⁺ concentration near the cell membrane is sufficiently raised due to the opening of receptor-gated or store-operated channels, the NCX may act in *reverse mode*, thereby becoming a pathway for Ca^{2+} influx rather than extrusion.

Most vasodilators acting on smooth muscle cells cause relaxation by activating either the **cyclic GMP** (e.g. nitric oxide, atrial natriuretic peptide) or **cyclic AMP** (e.g. adenosine, prostacyclin, β-receptor agonists) second messenger systems. Both second messengers activate kinases, which act by phosphorylating overlapping sets of cellular proteins. cGMP activates **cyclic GMP-dependent protein kinase (protein kinase G, PKG)**. PKG has multiple vasodilating effects. It activates K⁺ channels by phosphorylating them, leading to a membrane hyperpolarization that inhibits Ca^{2+} influx by switching off voltage-gated Ca^{2+} channels, a fraction of which are open even at the resting membrane potential. PKG also stimulates the sequestration and extrusion of Ca^{2+} sequestration by activating the Ca^{2+} pumps, and it stimulates myosin phophatase by inhibiting Rho kinase.

Cyclic AMP exerts its effects via **cyclic AMP-dependent protein kinase (protein kinase A, PKA)**, although high levels of cAMP have also been shown to stimulate PKG. PKA lowers $[Ca^{2+}]_i$ by stimulating Ca^{2+} pumps, and also by opening K⁺ channels (again via phosphorylation). The stimulation of SERCA by PKA, which loads the SR with Ca^{2+}, may also indirectly activate **Ca²⁺-activated K⁺ (BK_Ca) channels** by increasing the frequency of 'Ca²⁺ sparks'. These are transient elevations of $[Ca^{2+}]_i$ near the cell membrane caused by the opening of ryanodine receptors (RyRs) and the consequent release of Ca^{2+} from the SR. PKA can also phosphorylate MLCK, thereby inhibiting its activity. However, the contribution of this mechanism to relaxation under physiological conditions is controversial.

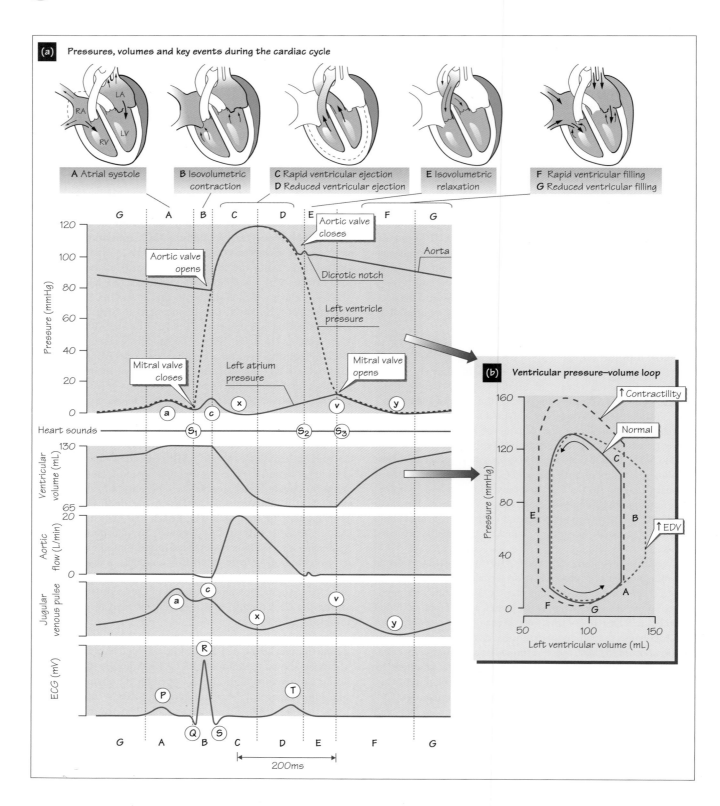

The Cardiovascular System at a Glance, Fourth Edition. Philip I. Aaronson, Jeremy P.T. Ward, and Michelle J. Connolly.

The **cardiac cycle** is the sequence of events that occurs during a heart beat (Figure 16a). The amount of blood ejected by the ventricle in this process is the **stroke volume** (SV), ~70 mL, and **cardiac output** is the volume ejected per minute (SV × heart rate).

Towards the end of **diastole** (G) all chambers of the heart are relaxed. The valves between the atria and ventricles are open (**AV valves**: right, **tricuspid**; left, **mitral**), because atrial pressure remains slightly greater than ventricular pressure until the ventricles are fully distended. The **pulmonary** and **aortic** (semilunar) **outflow valves** are closed, as pulmonary artery and aortic pressure are greater than the respective ventricular pressures. The cycle begins when the **sinoatrial node** initiates the heart beat (see Chapter 11).

Atrial systole (A)

Contraction of the atria completes ventricular filling. At rest, the atria contribute less than 20% of ventricular volume, but this proportion increases with heart rate, as diastole shortens and there is less time for ventricular filling. There are no valves between the veins and atria, and some blood regurgitates into the veins. The **a wave** of atrial and venous pressure traces reflects atrial systole. Ventricular volume after filling is known as **end-diastolic volume** (EDV), and is ~120–140 mL. The equivalent pressure (**end-diastolic pressure**, EDP) is <10 mmHg, and is higher in the left ventricle than in the right due to the more muscular and therefore stiffer left ventricular wall. EDV is an important determinant of the strength of the subsequent contraction (Starling's law; see Chapter 17). Atrial depolarization causes the **P wave** of the ECG.

Ventricular systole

Ventricular contraction causes a sharp rise in ventricular pressure, and the atrioventricular (AV) valves close once this exceeds atrial pressure. Closure of the AV valves causes the **first heart sound** (S_1; see below). Ventricular depolarization is associated with the **QRS complex** of the ECG. During the initial phase of ventricular contraction pressure is less than that in the pulmonary artery and aorta, so the outflow valves remain closed. This is **isovolumetric contraction** (B), as ventricular volume does not change. The increasing pressure causes the AV valves to bulge into the atria, resulting in the small atrial pressure wave (**c wave**), followed by a fall (**x descent**). Note the **jugular venous pulse** reflects the right atrial pressure, and has corresponding **a, c** and **v waves**, and **x** and **y descents**.

Ejection

The outflow valves open when pressure in the ventricle exceeds that in its respective artery. Note that pulmonary artery pressure (~15 mmHg) is considerably less than that in the aorta (~80 mmHg). Flow into the arteries is initially very rapid (**rapid ejection phase**, C), but as contraction wanes ejection is reduced (**reduced ejection phase**, D). Rapid ejection can sometimes be heard as a **murmur**. Active contraction ceases during the second half of ejection, and the muscle repolarizes. This is associated with the **T wave** of the ECG. Ventricular pressure towards the end of the reduced ejection phase is slightly less than that in the artery, but blood continues to flow out of the ventricle because of momentum. Eventually the flow briefly reverses, causing closure of the outflow valve and a small increase in aortic pressure, the **dicrotic notch**. Closure of the semilunar valves is associated with the second heart sound (S_2).

The ventricle ejects ~70 mL of blood (SV), so if EDV is 120 mL, 50 mL is left in the ventricle at the end of systole (**end-systolic volume**). The proportion of EDV that is ejected (stroke volume/EDV) is the **ejection fraction**. During the last two-thirds of systole atrial pressure rises as a result of filling from the veins (**v wave**).

Diastole – relaxation and refilling

Following closure of the outflow valves the ventricles are rapidly relaxing. Ventricular pressure is still greater than atrial pressure, however, and the AV valves remain closed. This is **isovolumetric relaxation** (E). When ventricular pressure falls below atrial pressure, the AV valves open, and atrial pressure falls (**y descent**) as the ventricles refill (**rapid ventricular refilling**, F). This is assisted by elastic recoil of the ventricular walls, essentially sucking in the blood. A **third heart sound** (S_3) may be heard. As the ventricles relax completely refilling slows (**reduced refilling**, G). This continues during the last two-thirds of diastole due to venous flow. At rest, diastole is twice the length of systole, but decreases proportionately during exercise and as heart rate increases.

The pressure–volume loop

Ventricular pressure plotted against volume generates a loop (Figure 16b). The shape of the loop is affected by **contractility** (see Chapters 12 and 17) and **compliance** ('*stretchiness*') of the ventricle, and factors that alter **refilling** or **ejection** (e.g. central venous pressure, afterload). The bottom dotted line shows the passive elastic properties of the ventricle (compliance). If compliance was decreased as a result of fibrotic damage following an infarct, the curve would be steeper. The area of the loop (Δ pressure × Δ volume) is a measure of work done during a beat, and is an indicator of cardiac function. A clinical estimate of **stroke work** is calculated from mean arterial pressure × stroke volume.

Heart sounds and murmurs

Heart sounds are caused by **vibrations in the blood**. S_1 and S_2 are each formed of two components (one for each valve). Normally, these may not be distinguishable, but they can 'split', so two distinct sounds are heard. S_1 is comprised of M_1 and T_1, due to closure of the mitral and tricuspid valves, respectively. Splitting of S_1 is always pathological, and commonly due to conduction defects (see Chapter 13). S_2 is comprised of A_2 and P_2, closure of aortic and pulmonary valves, respectively. A_2 slightly precedes P_2, and a split is often heard in healthy young people, especially during inspiration and exercise. A large split may relate to conduction defects or high outflow pressures. S_3 is due to rapid ventricular filling, and is often heard in young healthy people and also when EDP is high (e.g. heart failure). S_4 (not shown) is associated with atrial systole, and rarely heard unless EDP is high.

Murmurs are caused by turbulence. **Valve stenosis** (narrowing; see Chapter 52) increases blood velocity and thus turbulence. Stenosis of the AV valves causes a soft **diastolic murmur** during ventricular filling. Semilunar valve stenosis causes a loud **systolic murmur** during ejection. Valve leakage (**regurgitation**, *incompetence*) also causes murmurs. AV valve regurgitation causes a **pansystolic** murmur (throughout systole) as blood leaks back into the atria, whereas semilunar valve regurgitation causes **early diastolic** murmurs as arterial blood leaks back into the ventricle.

17 Control of cardiac output

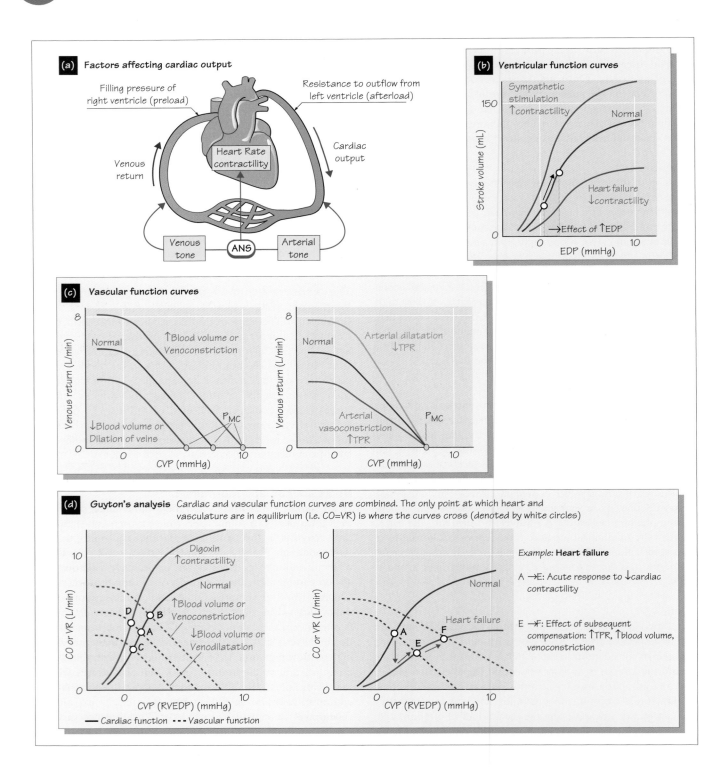

The Cardiovascular System at a Glance, Fourth Edition. Philip I. Aaronson, Jeremy P.T. Ward, and Michelle J. Connolly.

Cardiac output (CO) is stroke volume (SV) × heart rate (HR), and at rest ~5 L/min; during strenuous exercise this can rise to >25 L/min. SV is influenced by the filling pressure (**preload**), cardiac muscle force, and pressure against which the heart has to pump (**afterload**), which are all modulated by the autonomic nervous system (ANS) (Figure 17a). The heart and vasculature are in series and *interdependent*; except for transient differences **venous return** *must* equal CO.

Ventricular function curves

The volume of blood in the ventricle at the start of systole (**end-diastolic volume**, EDV) depends on the **end-diastolic pressure** (EDP) and **compliance** of the ventricular wall (how easy it is to inflate). Right ventricular (RV) EDP is dependent on **right atrial** and thus **central venous pressure** (CVP). If EDP (and so EDV) is increased, the force of the following contraction, and thus SV, increases (Figure 17b). This is known as the **Frank–Starling** relationship, and the graph relating SV to EDP is the **ventricular function** curve. The force of contraction is dependent on muscle stretch, and **Starling's law of the heart** states 'The energy released during contraction depends on the initial fibre length.'

As muscle is stretched, more myosin crossbridges can form, increasing force. Cardiac muscle has a steeper relationship between stretch and force than skeletal muscle, because in the heart stretch also increases Ca^{2+} binding to troponin C (see Chapter 12). The function curve is therefore steep, so small changes in EDP can lead to large increases in SV and CO (Figure 17b).

Role of Starling's law

The most important consequence of Starling's law is that **output is matched between right and left ventricles**. If, for example, RV SV increases, the amount of blood in the lungs and thus pulmonary vascular pressure must also increase. As the latter determines left ventricular (LV) EDP, LV SV increases due to Starling's law, until it again matches RV SV when input to and output from the lungs equalize and the pressure stops rising. This represents a rightward shift along the function curve (Figure 17b). Starling's law thus explains how CVP, although only perceived by the RV, also influences LV function and CO, and why postural hypotension and haemorrhage reduce CO. It also allows the heart to sustain output when afterload is increased (hypertension, valve stenosis) or *contractility* reduced (e.g. heart failure; Figure 17b; see Chapter 46), as both lead to accumulation of venous blood and a raised EDP, which increases ventricular force and restores SV. Note that any increase in LV EDP represents an increase in RV afterload, so for the same reasons CVP may also rise (Figure 17d). As EDV is necessarily increased in the above cases, **ejection fraction** (SV/EDV) will be reduced; a greatly reduced ejection fraction and **enlarged heart** (high EDV) are diagnostic for systolic heart failure (see Chapter 46).

The autonomic nervous system

The ANS strongly influences CO, and is central to control of blood pressure (see Chapters 27 and 28). **Sympathetic** stimulation increases heart rate and cardiac muscle force (see Chapters 11 and 12). Force is increased *without any change in EDP* (i.e. increased stretch), so that the function curve is shifted upwards (Figure 17b). This is called an increase in **contractility**, and agents that affect contractility are called **inotropes** (see Chapter 12). **Parasympathetic**

stimulation slows the heart but does not decrease contractility, as ventricular parasympathetic innervation is sparse.

Activation of sympathetic nerves also causes arterial and venous vasoconstriction (see Chapter 28). An important but often overlooked point is that these differ in effect. Arterial vasoconstriction increases total peripheral resistance (TPR) and thus reduces flow, so downstream pressure and venous return will fall. However, the veins contain ~70% of the blood volume at low pressure and are highly **compliant** (stretch easily). Venoconstriction does not significantly impede flow because their resistance is low compared to arteries, but it reduces their **compliance** and hence **capacity** (amount of blood they contain). Thus, venoconstriction has the same effect as increasing blood volume, and **increases CVP**. Sympathetic stimulation can thus increase CO by increasing heart rate, contractility and CVP.

Vascular function curves and Guyton's analysis

The **vascular function curve** depicts the relationship between venous return and CVP (Figure 17c). Blood flow is driven by the arterial–venous pressure difference, so **venous return** will be impeded by a rise in CVP. If the heart stops, pressure will equalize between the arterial and venous circulations (**mean circulatory pressure, P_{MC}**), which depends on the volume and compliance of the vasculature, primarily the veins (see above). By definition CVP equals P_{MC} when venous return (i.e. CO) is zero. The curve levels off at negative CVP due to venous collapse. Raising blood volume or venoconstriction increases P_{MC} and so causes a parallel shift of the curve to the right, whereas blood loss does the reverse. Arterial vasoconstriction and an increase in TPR on the other hand reduces blood flow and venous return at any CVP (see above), but as resistance arteries contain little of the blood volume, and the decrease in diameter required to increase their resistance is small (see Chapter 18), there is an insignificant change in vascular volume or P_{MC}. Thus, the net effect is to reduce the slope of the curve. A reduction in TPR does the opposite.

Guyton's analysis helps us to understand the integrated function of the cardiovascular system by combining vascular and cardiac function curves into one graph (Figure 17d). The cardiac function curve is now shown as CO plotted against CVP (i.e. RV EDP). The only point at which CO and venous return are equal, and so the only point where the system is in equilibrium, is where the two function curves cross (A), the **equilibrium** (or *operating*) point. Thus, **increasing blood volume** or **venoconstriction** shifts the equilibrium point (B) and CO and CVP are both increased. Blood loss or venous dilatation do the opposite (C), which is why nitrovasodilators, which primarily dilate veins, reduce cardiac work (see Chapter 41). **Positive inotropes** (e.g. digoxin) increase cardiac contractility and shift the cardiac function curve upwards. At equilibrium (D) CO is thus increased but CVP *reduced*, explaining why digoxin reduces symptoms in heart failure (but not survival; see Chapter 46). Analysis of **heart failure** is illuminating. The initial fall in CO is limited by an elevated CVP (Figure 17d, E; see Starling's law above). Central mechanisms mediated via the ANS then provide further compensation against a fall in blood pressure, by increasing TPR, venoconstriction and renal retention of salt and water (see Chapter 46). Combined, these raise and flatten the vascular function curve (see above), so at equilibrium CO may be largely restored, but at the expense of a greatly increased CVP (F).

18 Haemodynamics

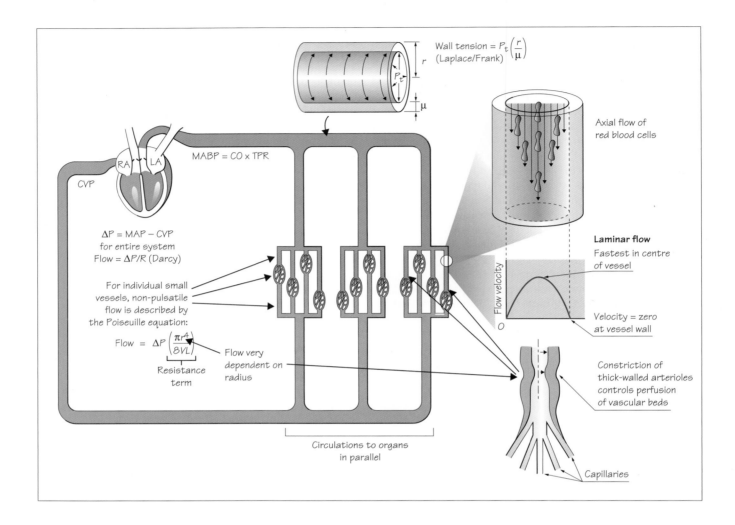

Wall tension $= P_t\left(\dfrac{r}{\mu}\right)$ (Laplace/Frank)

Axial flow of red blood cells

MABP = CO × TPR

ΔP = MAP – CVP
for entire system
Flow = $\Delta P/R$ (Darcy)

For individual small vessels, non-pulsatile flow is described by the Poiseuille equation:

Flow $= \Delta P\left(\dfrac{\pi r^4}{8VL}\right)$

Flow very dependent on radius

Resistance term

Circulations to organs in parallel

Laminar flow
Fastest in centre of vessel

Velocity = zero at vessel wall

Constriction of thick-walled arterioles controls perfusion of vascular beds

Capillaries

Relationships between pressure, resistance and flow

Haemodynamics is the study of the relationships between **pressure**, **resistance** and the **flow of blood** in the cardiovascular system. Although the properties of this flow are enormously complex, they can largely be derived from simpler physical laws governing the flow of liquids through single tubes.

When a fluid is pumped through a closed system, its flow (Q) is determined by the pressure head developed by the pump (P_1-P_2 or ΔP), and by the resistance (R) to that flow, according to **Darcy's law** (analogous to Ohm's law):

$$Q = \Delta P/R$$

or for the cardiovascular system as a whole:

$$CO = (MABP - CVP)/TPR,$$

where CO is cardiac output, $MABP$ is mean arterial blood pressure, TPR is total peripheral resistance and CVP is central venous pressure. Because CVP is ordinarily close to zero, $MABP$ is equal to $CO \times TPR$.

Resistance to flow is caused by frictional forces within the fluid, and depends on the viscosity of the fluid and the dimensions of the tube, as described by **Poiseuille's law**:

$$resistance = 8VL/\pi r^4$$

so that:

$$flow = \Delta P(\pi r^4/8VL).$$

Here, V is the viscosity of the fluid, L is the tube length and r is the inner radius (= $^1/2$ the diameter) of the tube. Because flow depends on the 4th power of the tube radius in this equation, *small changes in radius have a powerful effect on flow*. For example, a 20% decrease in radius reduces flow by about 60%.

Considering the cardiovascular system as a whole, the different types or sizes of blood vessels (e.g. arteries, arterioles, capillaries) are arranged sequentially, or in *series*. In this case, the resistance of the entire system is equal to the *sum of all the resistances* offered by each type of vessel:

$$R_{total} = R_{arteries} + R_{arterioles} + R_{capillaries} + R_{venules} + R_{veins}.$$

The Cardiovascular System at a Glance, Fourth Edition. Philip I. Aaronson, Jeremy P.T. Ward, and Michelle J. Connolly.

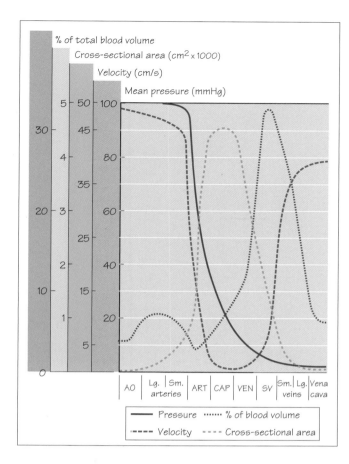

% of total blood volume
Cross-sectional area (cm² x 1000)
Velocity (cm/s)
Mean pressure (mmHg)

AO | Lg. Sm. arteries | ART | CAP | VEN | SV | Sm. Lg. veins | Vena cava

—— Pressure ⋯⋯ % of blood volume
---- Velocity ---- Cross-sectional area

Calculations taking into account the estimated lengths, radii and numbers of the various sizes of blood vessels show that the arterioles, and to a lesser extent the capillaries and venules, are primarily responsible for the resistance of the cardiovascular system to the flow of blood. In other words, $R_{\text{arteriole}}$ makes the largest contribution to R_{total}. Because according to Darcy's law the pressure drop in any section of the system is proportional to the resistance of that section, the steepest fall in pressure is in the arterioles (Figure 18.2).

Although the various sizes of blood vessel are arranged in series, each organ or region of the body is supplied by its own major arteries which emerge from the aorta. The vascular beds for the various organs are therefore arranged in *parallel* with each other. Similarly, the vascular beds within each organ are mainly arranged into parallel subdivisions (e.g. the arteriolar resistances $R_{\text{arteriole}}$ are in parallel with each other). For 'n' vascular beds arranged in parallel:

$$1/R_{\text{total}} = 1/R_1 + 1/R_2 + 1/R_3 + 1/R_4 \ldots 1/R_n.$$

An important consequence of this relationship is that the blood flow to a particular organ can be altered (by adjustments of the resistances of the arterioles in that organ) without greatly affecting pressures and flows in the rest of the system. This can be accom-

plished, as a consequence of Poiseuille's law, by relatively small dilatations or constrictions of the arterioles within an organ or vascular bed.

Because there are so many small blood vessels (e.g. millions of arterioles, billions of venules, trillions of capillaries), the overall cross-sectional area of the vasculature reaches its peak in the microcirculation. As the velocity of the blood at any level in the system is equal to the total flow (the cardiac output) divided by the cross-sectional area at that level, the blood flow is slowest in the capillaries (Figure 18.2), favouring O_2–CO_2 exchange and tissue absorption of nutrients. The capillary transit time at rest is 0.5–2 s.

Blood viscosity

Very viscous fluids like motor oil flow more slowly than less viscous fluids like water. **Viscosity** is caused by frictional forces within a fluid that resist flow. Although the viscosity of plasma is similar to that of water, the viscosity of blood is normally three to four times that of water, because of the presence of blood cells, mainly erythrocytes. In **anaemia**, where the cell concentration (haematocrit) is low, viscosity and therefore vascular resistance decrease, and CO rises. Conversely, in the high-haematocrit condition **polycythaemia**, vascular resistance and blood pressure are increased.

Laminar flow

As liquid flows steadily through a long tube, frictional forces are exerted by the tube wall. These, in addition to viscous forces within the liquid, set up a velocity gradient across the tube (Figure 18.1) in which the fluid adjacent to the wall is motionless, and the flow velocity is greatest at the centre of the tube. This is termed **laminar flow**, and occurs in the microcirculation, except in the smallest capillaries. One consequence of laminar flow is that erythrocytes tend to move away from the vessel wall and align themselves edgewise in the flow stream. This reduces the effective viscosity of the blood in the microcirculation (the **Fåhraeus–Lindqvist effect**), helping to minimize resistance.

Wall tension

In addition to the pressure gradient along the length of blood vessels, there exists a pressure difference across the wall of a blood vessel. This transmural pressure is equal to the pressure inside the vessel minus the interstitial pressure. The transmural pressure exerts a circumferential tension on the wall of the blood vessel that tends to distend it, much as high pressure within a balloon stretches it. According to the **Laplace/Frank law**:

$$\text{wall tension} = P_t(r/\mu),$$

where P_t is the transmural pressure, r is the vessel radius and μ is the wall thickness. In the aorta, where P_t and r are high, atherosclerosis may cause thinning of the arterial wall and the development of a bulge or **aneurysm** (see Chapter 37). This increases r and decreases μ, setting up a vicious cycle of increasing wall tension which, if not treated, may result in vessel rupture.

Blood pressure and flow in the arteries and arterioles

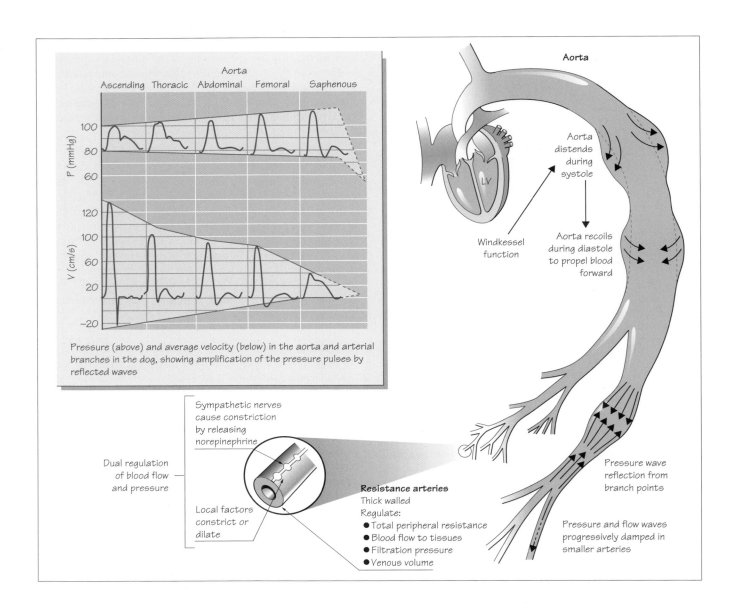

Pressure (above) and average velocity (below) in the aorta and arterial branches in the dog, showing amplification of the pressure pulses by reflected waves

Factors controlling arterial blood pressure

The mean arterial blood pressure is equal to the product of the cardiac output (about 5 L/min at rest) and the total peripheral resistance (TPR). Because the total drop of mean pressure across the systemic circulation is about 100 mmHg, TPR is calculated to be 100 mmHg/5000 mL/min, or 0.02 mmHg/mL/min. The unit mmHg/mL/min is referred to as a **peripheral resistance unit** (PRU), so that TPR is normally about 0.02 PRU.

Systolic pressure is mainly influenced by the *stroke volume*, the *left ventricular ejection velocity* and *aortic/arterial stiffness*, and rises when any of these increase. Conversely, diastolic pressure rises with an *increase in TPR*. Arterial pressure falls progressively during diastole (see Figure 16), so that a shortening of the diastolic

interval associated with a rise in the heart rate also increases diastolic pressure.

Blood pressure and flow in the arteries

The blood flow in the aorta and the larger arteries is pulsatile, as a result of the rhythmic emptying of the left ventricle.

As blood is ejected from the left ventricle during systole, it hits the column of blood already present in the ascending aorta, creating a pressure wave in the aortic blood which is rapidly (at between 4 and 10 m/s) conducted towards the arterioles. As this pulse pressure wave passes each point along the aorta and the major arteries, it sets up a transient pressure gradient that briefly propels the blood at that point forward, causing a pulsatile flow wave. The blood in the arteries therefore moves forward in short bursts, separated by longer periods of stasis, so that its average velocity in the aorta is about 0.2 m/s.

The pressure wave also causes the elastic arterial wall to bulge out, thereby storing some of the energy of the wave. The arterial wall then rebounds, releasing part of this energy to drive the blood forward during diastole (**diastolic run-off**). This pumping mechanism of the elastic arteries is termed the **Windkessel** function (Figure 19).

The large arteries also absorb and dissipate some of the energy of the pressure wave. This progressively damps the oscillations in flow, as shown by the lower traces in the inset to Figure 19. However, as the upper traces illustrate, the pulse pressure wave becomes somewhat *larger* as it moves down the aorta and major arteries (e.g. the saphenous artery), before it then progressively dies out along the smaller arteries. This occurs in part because a fraction of the pressure wave is *reflected* back towards the heart at arterial branch points. In the aorta and large arteries, the reflected wave *summates* with the forward-moving pulse pressure wave, increasing its amplitude. Once the blood has entered the smaller arteries, however, the damping properties of the arterial wall predominate, and progressively depress the oscillations in flow and pressure, so that these die out completely by the time the blood reaches the microcirculation.

Arterioles and vascular resistance

The mean blood pressure falls progressively along the arterial system. The decline is particularly steep in the smallest arteries and the arterioles (diameter <100 μm), because these vessels present the greatest resistance to flow (Figure 18.2). The walls of the arterioles are very thick in relation to the diameter of the lumen, and these vessels can therefore constrict powerfully, dramatically increasing this resistance. Because the arterioles are normally partially constricted, their resistance can also be decreased by vasodilating stimuli.

The role of the arterioles in setting the vascular resistance has several important implications.

1 Constriction or dilatation of all, or a large proportion, of the arterioles in the body will affect the TPR and the blood pressure.

2 Constriction of the arterioles in one organ or region will selectively direct the flow of blood away from that region, while dilatation will have the opposite effect.

3 Changes in arteriolar resistance in a region affect the 'downstream' hydrostatic pressure within the capillary beds and veins in that region. Changes in the pressure within the capillaries affect the movement of fluid from the blood to the tissues (see Chapter 21). Because the veins are very compliant, their volume is very sensitive to alterations in pressure (see Chapter 22). Thus, arteriolar constriction in a region of the body will both promote the movement of fluid from its tissue spaces into its exchange vessels, and also decrease its venous volume. Both effects work to increase the blood supply to other parts of the body.

Table 19.1 lists important endogenous substances and factors that affect arteriolar tone.

Table 19.1 Endogenous substances and other factors affecting arteriolar tone.

	Vasoconstrictors	Vasodilators

Neurotransmitters	Sympathetic
	    Noradrenaline
	ATP
	Neuropeptide Y
		Parasympathetic and sensory (limited distribution)
		    Acetylcholine (acts via NO)
		Substance P
		Calcitonin gene-related peptide
		Vasoactive intestinal peptide

Hormones	Adrenaline (most blood vessels) Angiotensin II Vasopressin (antidiuretic hormone)	Adrenaline (in skeletal muscle, coronary, hepatic arteries) Atrial natriuretic peptide

Endothelium-
    derived
    substances
	Endothelin
	Endothelium-derived constricting
	    factor (chemical identity unknown)
		Endothelium-derived relaxing factor (NO)
		Prostaglandin I_2 (prostacyclin)

Metabolites and
    related factors
	Hypoxia (pulmonary arteries only)	Endothelium-derived hyperpolarizing factor (chemical identity
		    unknown)
		Hypoxia (other vessels)
		Adenosine, hyperosmolarity, H^+ ions, lactic acid, K^+ ions, CO_2

Other locally
    produced
    factors
	Histamine (veins, pulmonary arteries)
	Prostaglandin $F_{2\alpha}$, thromboxane A_2
	5-Hydroxytryptamine
	Growth factors (e.g. PDGF)
		Histamine (arterioles)
		Prostaglandin E_2
		Bradykinin

Other factors	Pressure (myogenic response) Moderate cold (skin)	Increased flow Heat (skin)

NO, nitric oxide; PDGF, platelet-derived growth factor.

The microcirculation and lymphatic system, and diapedesis

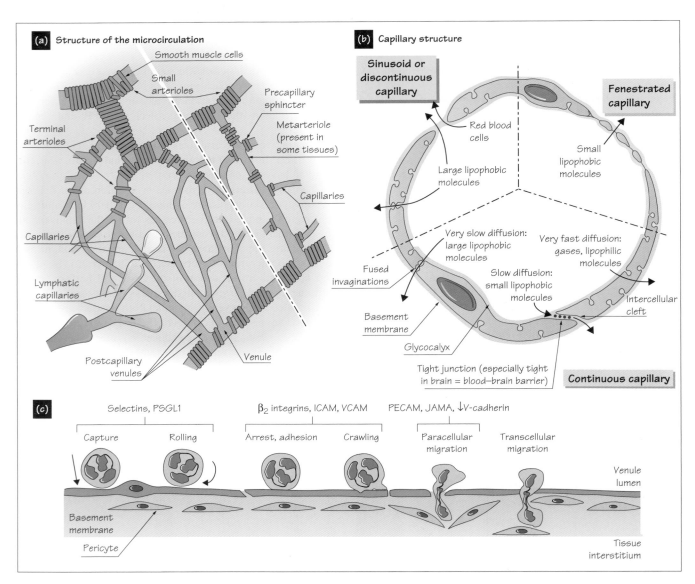

The **microcirculation** comprises the **smallest arterioles**, and the **exchange vessels**, including the **capillaries** and the **postcapillary venules**. The transfer of gases, water, nutrients, waste materials and other substances between the blood and body tissues carried out by the exchange vessels is the ultimate function of the cardiovascular system.

Organization of the microcirculation

Blood enters the microcirculation via small arterioles, the walls of which contain smooth muscle cells. These vessels are densely innervated by the sympathetic system, particularly in the splanchnic and cutaneous vascular beds. Sympathetically mediated constriction of each small arteriole reduces the blood flow to many capillaries.

In the vast majority of tissues, the smallest or **terminal** arterioles divide to give rise to sets of capillaries (Figure 20a, left). The terminal arteriole itself acts as a functional precapillary sphincter for

its entire cluster of capillaries. Terminal arterioles are not innervated, and their tone is controlled by local metabolic factors (see Chapter 23). Under basal conditions, terminal arterioles constrict and relax periodically. This **vasomotion** causes the flow of blood through the cluster of capillaries to fluctuate.

In a few tissues, however (e.g. mesentery), capillaries branch from thoroughfare vessels which run from small arterioles to venules (Figure 20a, right). The proximal (arteriolar) end of such a vessel is termed a **metarteriole**, and it is wrapped intermittently in smooth muscle cells. The capillaries have a ring of smooth muscle called a **precapillary sphincter** at their origin, but thereafter lack smooth muscle cells. Constriction of the precapillary sphincter controls the flow of blood through that capillary.

The capillaries join to form postcapillary venules, which also lack smooth muscle cells. These merge to form venules, which contain smooth muscle cells and are sympathetically innervated.

The Cardiovascular System at a Glance, Fourth Edition. Philip I. Aaronson, Jeremy P.T. Ward, and Michelle J. Connolly.

Movement of solutes across the capillary wall

Water, gases and solutes (e.g. electrolytes, glucose, proteins) cross the walls of exchange vessels mainly by **diffusion**, a passive process by which substances move down their concentration gradients. O_2 and CO_2 can diffuse through the lipid bilayers of the endothelial cells. These and other **lipophilic** substances (e.g. general anaesthetics) therefore cross the capillary wall very rapidly. However, the lipid bilayer is impermeable to electrolytes and small **hydrophilic** (lipid-insoluble) molecules such as glucose, which therefore cross the walls of **continuous** capillaries (Figure 20b, bottom) 1000–10000 times more slowly than does O_2. Hydrophilic molecules cross the capillary wall mainly by diffusing between the endothelial cells. This process is slowed by tight junctions between the endothelial cells which impede diffusion through the intercellular clefts. Diffusion is also retarded by the **glycocalyx**, a dense network of fibrous macromolecules coating the luminal side of the endothelium. This tortuous diffusion pathway (the **small pore system**) acts as a sieve which admits molecules of molecular weight (MW) less than 10000.

Even large proteins (e.g. albumin, MW 69000) can cross the capillary wall, albeit very slowly. This suggests that the capillary wall also contains a small number of **large pores**, although these have never been directly visualized. It has been proposed that large pores exist transiently when membrane invaginations on either side of the endothelial cell fuse, temporarily creating a channel through which large molecules diffuse.

The endothelial cells of **fenestrated** capillaries (found in kidneys, intestines and joints) contain pores called **fenestrae** (Figure 20b, upper right) which render them ~10 times more permeable than continuous capillaries to small hydrophilic molecules, which can move through the fenestrae. **Sinusoidal** or **discontinuous** capillaries (liver, bone marrow, spleen) are very highly permeable, because they have wide spaces between adjacent endothelial cells through which proteins and even erythrocytes can pass (Figure 20b, upper left).

The blood–brain barrier

The composition of the extracellular fluid in the brain must be kept extremely constant in order to allow stable neuronal function. This is made possible by the existence of the **blood–brain barrier** (BBB), which tightly controls the movement of ions and solutes across the walls of the continuous capillaries within the brain and the choroid plexus. The BBB has two important features. First, the junctions between the endothelial cells of cerebral capillaries are extremely tight (resembling the zonae occludens of epithelia), preventing any significant movement of hydrophilic solutes. Second, specialized membrane transporters exist in cerebral endothelial cells which allow the controlled movement of inorganic ions, glucose, amino acids and other substances across the capillary wall. Thus, the relatively uncontrolled diffusion of solutes present in other vascular beds is replaced in the brain by a number of specific transport processes. This can present a therapeutic problem, as most drugs are excluded from the brain (e.g. many antibiotics).

The BBB is interrupted in the **circumventricular organs**, areas of the brain that need to be influenced by blood-borne factors, or to release substances into the blood. These include the **pituitary** and **pineal** glands, the **median eminence**, the **area postrema** and the **choroid plexus**. The BBB can break down with large elevations of blood pressure, osmolarity or P_{CO_2}, and in infected areas of the brain.

Diapedesis

In order to cause local inflammation in infected or damaged tissue, leucocytes must leave the blood by migrating across the endothelium of nearby venules, a process termed **diapedesis** (Figure 20c). Inflammatory mediators released at the site of infection induce venular endothelial cells to express E- and P-selectins and other adhesion molecules on their luminal surfaces. Leucocytes express complementary surface adhesion molecules such as VLA_4 and P-selectin glycoprotein ligand 1, and many leucocytes are therefore captured as they flow by, at first rolling along the endothelial surface and then stopping as their interaction with the endothelium and exposure to locally released cytokines causes the expression and activation of additional adhesion molecules on both types of cells (e.g. VCAM1 on endothelial cells; β_2 integrins on leucocytes). The leucocytes flatten and send out protrusions allowing them to creep over the endothelium, seeking 'permissive' sites at which they can enter the tissue by squeezing themselves through the junctions *between* adjacent endothelial cells (**paracellular transendothelial migration**). Endothelial cells aid this process by down-regulating the function of the junctional plasmalemmal protein VE-cadherin which normally acts to hold the adjacent cells close together at the junctions, and by transiently increasing the expression of junctional adhesion molecules such as PECAM and JAM-A, which the leucocytes use to pull themselves through. Alternatively, leucocytes are able to undergo **transcellular transendothelial migration**, a process by which they tunnel directly *through* rather than between endothelial cells to reach the interstitium. Following endothelial transmigration, leucocytes are able to propel themselves through weak spots in the layer of basement membrane and pericytes, gaining access to the tissue.

The lymphatic system

Approximately 8 L of fluid containing solutes and plasma proteins is filtered from the microcirculation into the tissue spaces each day. This returns to the blood via the **lymphatic system**. Most body tissues contain lymphatic capillaries (Figure 20a). These are blind-ended bulbous tubes 15–75 μm in diameter, with walls formed of a monolayer of endothelial cells. Interstitial fluid, plasma proteins and bacteria can easily enter the lymphatic capillaries via the gaps between these cells, the arrangement of which then prevents these substances from escaping. These vessels merge to form **collecting lymphatics**, the walls of which contain smooth muscle cells and one-way valves (as do the larger lymphatic vessels). The sections between these valves constrict strongly, forcing the lymph towards the blood. Lymph is also propelled by compression of the vessels by muscular contraction, body movement and tissue compression. Lymph then enters the larger **afferent lymphatics**, which flow into the **lymph nodes**. Here, foreign particles and bacteria are scavenged by phagocytes, and can initiate the production of activated lymphocytes. These enter the lymph for transport into the circulation, where they mount an immune response. Much of the lymph returns to the blood via capillary absorption in the lymph nodes. The rest enters **efferent lymphatics**, most of which eventually merge into the **thoracic duct**. This duct empties into the left subclavian vein in the neck. Lymphatics from parts of the thorax, the right arm and the right sides of the head and neck merge forming the **right lymph duct**, which enters the right subclavian vein. The lymphatic system is also important in the absorption of lipids from the intestines. The **lacteal** lymphatics are responsible for transporting about 60% of digested fat into the venous blood.

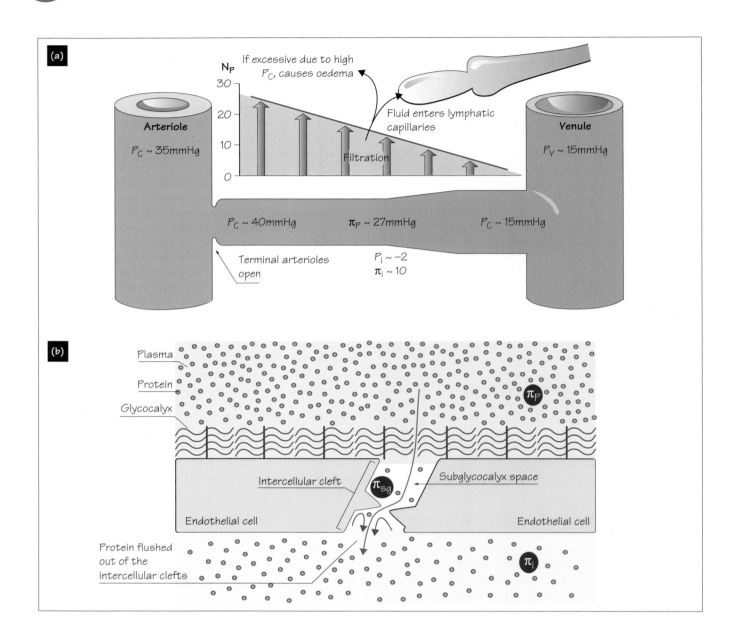

Movement of water across the capillary wall

The capillary wall (here taken to include the wall of postcapillary venules) is very permeable to water. However, although individual water molecules can move freely between the plasma and the tissue spaces, the *net* flow of water across the capillary wall is very small. This flow is determined by a balance between two forces or pressures that are exerted across the wall of the capillaries. These are **hydrostatic pressure**, which tends to drive water out of the capillary, and **colloid osmotic pressure**, which tends to draw water into capillaries from the surrounding tissue spaces. The sum of these two pressures at each point along the capillary is equal to a net pressure that will be directed either out of or into the capillary, and the net flow of water is proportional to this net pressure. The classic **Starling equation** describes the relationship between net flow (J_v) and the hydrostatic and osmotic pressures:

$$J_v \propto [(P_c - P_i) - \sigma(\pi_p - \pi_i)]$$

The **hydrostatic force** ($P_c - P_i$) is equal to the difference between the blood pressure inside the capillary (P_c) and the pressure in the interstitium around the capillary (P_i). P_c in blood-perfused capillaries ranges from about 35 mmHg at the arteriolar end of the capillaries to about 15 mmHg in the venules. P_i is slightly subatmospheric in many tissues (−5 to 0 mmHg), due to a suction of fluid from the interstitium by the lymphatic capillaries. The greater

The Cardiovascular System at a Glance, Fourth Edition. Philip I. Aaronson, Jeremy P.T. Ward, and Michelle J. Connolly.

pressure inside the capillary tends to drive **filtration**, the movement of water out into the tissues.

As described in Chapter 20, the capillary wall acts as a *semipermeable membrane* or barrier to free diffusion, across which electrolytes and small molecules pass with much greater ease than plasma proteins. A substance dissolved on one side of a semipermeable membrane exerts an osmotic pressure that draws water across the membrane from the other side. This osmotic pressure is proportional to the concentration of the substance in solution, and is also a function of its permeability. Substances that can easily permeate a barrier (in this case the capillary wall) exert little osmotic pressure across it, whereas those that permeate less readily exert a larger osmotic pressure. For this reason, the osmotic force across the capillary wall is largely a result of the relatively impermeant plasma proteins, in particular albumin. The osmotic pressure exerted by plasma proteins is referred to as the **colloid osmotic** or **oncotic** pressure.

The osmotic force across the capillary wall tends to cause **absorption**, the movement of water into capillaries. This force has classically been equated with the difference between the colloid osmotic pressure of the plasma (π_p) and that of the interstitium (π_i), multiplied by the **reflection coefficient** (σ), a factor that is a measure of how difficult it for the proteins to cross the capillary wall. Substances that cannot cross the membrane at all have a reflection coefficient of 1, while those that pass freely have a reflection coefficient of zero. σ ranges from 0.8 to 0.95 for most plasma proteins, while ($\pi_p - \pi_i$) is typically about 13 mmHg.

Water filtration and absorption

Given the balance of hydrostatic and osmotic pressures acting on fluid in the microcirculation, capillaries and venules that are perfused with blood will be mainly filtering plasma (Figure 21a), so that normally there is a slight predominance of filtration over absorption in the body as a whole. Therefore, of about 4000 L plasma entering the capillaries daily as the blood recirculates, a *net* filtration of 8 L occurs. This fluid is returned from the interstitium to the vascular compartment through the lymphatic system.

On the other hand, certain sites such as the kidneys or the intestinal mucosa are specialized for water reabsorption. Here the osmotic pressure term is large, because plasma proteins are continually being washed out of the interstitium, so that net reabsorption occurs.

It is also the case that the balance between filtration and reabsorption is a dynamic one, mainly because the hydrostatic pressure within the capillaries is variable. Arteriolar vasodilatation, which increases intracapillary hydrostatic pressure, increases filtration, while arteriolar vasoconstriction favours absorption. For example, arterioles often demonstrate **vasomotion** (i.e. random opening and closing). During periods of arteriolar constriction, capillary pressure falls, favouring the absorption of interstitial fluid. This absorption tends to be transient, however, because as fluid is absorbed into the capillaries, local P_i falls and π_i increases. These effects progressively diminish absorption.

Assumption of the upright posture increases the transcapillary hydrostatic pressure gradient in the lower extremities, thereby immediately increasing filtration in these regions. However, this effect is partially compensated for by a rapid constriction of the arterioles of the leg, which is mediated by a local sympathetic axon reflex. This reduces blood flow and attenuates the rise in capillary hydrostatic pressure in these areas.

By the same token, fluid tends to accumulate in the tissue spaces of the upper body and face during the night, because assumption of the supine position increases capillary hydrostatic pressures above the heart. This causes morning 'puffiness'.

Although the principle on which the Starling equation is based is universally accepted, studies in many types of tissue have shown that net filtration is less than would be predicted from measurements of π_i. This discrepancy is explained by the Michel – Weinbaum hypothesis (Figure 21). According to this proposal, the glycocalyx coating the luminal endothelial wall constitutes the semipermeable diffusion barrier described above. Because water crosses the endothelium mainly through the glycocalyx and intercellular clefts, it is not the osmotic pressure exerted by the [protein] in the tissue interstitium (π_i), but rather the osmotic pressure exerted by the [protein] *within the intracellular clefts just beneath the glycocalyx*, which should be used to calculate the osmotic force term in the Starling equation. Importantly, this 'subglycocalyx' protein concentration (π_{sg}) is lower than that in the bulk interstitium because as water streams out through the clefts, it is funnelled through narrow gaps in the junctional strands that hold the walls of the clefts together, creating a current that opposes the diffusion of interstitial protein into the cleft which also occurs through these gaps. Modifying the Starling equation by replacing π_i with π_{sg} increases the size of the osmotic term in the equation (i.e. $\sigma(\pi_p - \pi_{sg})$ is larger than $\sigma(\pi_p - \pi_i)$ because $\pi_{sg} < \pi_i$) meaning that net filtration will be smaller than is predicted by the classic Starling equation.

Pulmonary and systemic oedema

The hydrostatic and osmotic pressures in the capillaries of the pulmonary circulation are atypical. Both P_c (~7 mmHg) and P_i (~8 mmHg) are low, while π_i is high (~18 mmHg), because these vessels are highly permeable to plasma proteins. The balance of forces slightly favours filtration. In **congestive heart failure**, the output of both the left and right ventricles is markedly reduced (see Chapter 46). Failure of the left ventricle results in an increase in left ventricular end-diastolic pressure. This pressure backs up into the lungs, causing increased pulmonary venular and capillary pressures. This promotes filtration in these vessels, causing an accumulation of fluid in the lungs (**pulmonary oedema**), which dramatically worsens the dyspnoea (breathlessness) and inadequate tissue oxygenation characteristic of congestive heart failure. Similarly, failure of the right ventricle increases systemic venous and therefore capillary pressure, leading to systemic oedema, particularly of the lower extremities.

Oedema of the legs is also caused by **varicose veins**, a condition in which the venous valves are unable to operate properly because the veins become swollen and overstretched. By interfering with the effectiveness of the skeletal muscle pump, the incompetence of the valves leads to increases in venous and capillary hydrostatic pressure, resulting in the rapid development of oedema during standing.

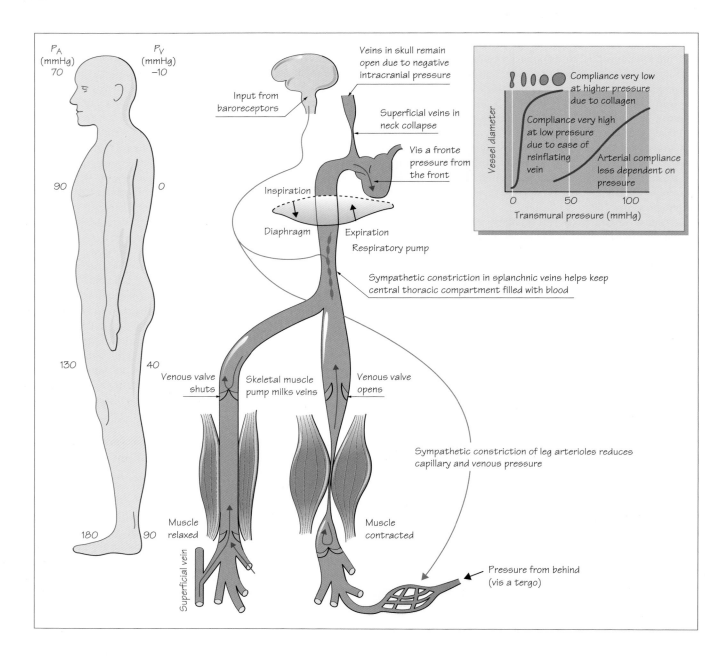

The venules and veins return the blood from the microcirculation to the right atrium. However, they do not serve merely as passive conduits. Instead, they have a crucial active role in stabilizing and regulating the **venous return** of blood to the heart.

The venous system differs from the arterial system in two important respects. First, the total volume (and cross-sectional area) of the venous system is much greater than that of the arterial system. This is because there are many more venules than arterioles; venules also tend to have larger internal diameters than arterioles. Second, the veins are quite thin walled, and can there-

fore expand greatly to hold more blood if their internal pressure rises.

As a result of its large cross-sectional area, the venous system offers much less resistance to flow than the arterial system. The pressure gradient required to drive the blood through the venous system (15 mmHg) is therefore much smaller than the pressure needed in the arterial system (80 mmHg). The average pressure in the venae cavae at the level of the heart (the **central venous pressure**) is usually close to 0 mmHg (i.e. atmospheric pressure). The flow of blood back to the heart is aided by the presence of one-way

The Cardiovascular System at a Glance, Fourth Edition. Philip I. Aaronson, Jeremy P.T. Ward, and Michelle J. Connolly.

venous valves in the arms and especially the legs, which prevent backflow.

Venous arterial compliance

The graph in Figure 22 (upper right) illustrates the relationship between pressure and volume in a typical vein and artery. The slope of the volume – pressure curve is referred to as the compliance. Compliance is a measure of expandability. Veins are much more compliant than arteries at low pressures (0–10 mmHg). Small increases in venous pressure in this range therefore cause large increases in venous blood volume.

One reason for high venous compliance is that their thin walls allow veins to collapse at low internal pressures. Only small increases in pressure are needed to 'reinflate' a collapsed vein with blood until it has nearly rounded up. At higher pressures, however, venous compliance decreases dramatically (see graph) because the slack in rigid collagen fibres in the venous wall is rapidly taken up. This limit on the expandability of the veins is important in limiting the pooling of blood in the veins of the legs that occurs during standing.

The veins as capacitance vessels

Because of their large volumes and high compliance, the veins/venules accommodate a much larger volume of the blood (~70% of the total) than do the arteries/arterioles (~12%). They are therefore termed capacitance vessels, and are able to serve as blood volume reservoirs. During exercise, and in hypotensive states (e.g. during haemorrhage), sympathetically mediated constriction of the veins/venules, notably in the splanchnic (including the gastrointestinal tract and liver) and cutaneous circulations, displaces blood into the rest of the cardiovascular system. In particular, the resulting reduction of the venous volume increases the volume of blood in the central thoracic compartment (i.e. the heart and pulmonary circulation), thereby boosting cardiac output, assisting perfusion of other essential vascular beds and helping to maintain the blood pressure.

Effects of posture

When the upright position is assumed, the pull of gravity increases the absolute pressures within *both* the arteries and veins of the lower extremities. The average arterial and venous blood pressures in a normal adult standing quietly are about 100 and 0 mmHg, respectively, at the level of the heart, while in the feet the pressures are about 190 and 90 mmHg, respectively. However, gravity does not affect the *pressure gradient* driving the blood circulation, because the *difference* between the arterial and venous pressures is similar (100 mmHg) at both levels. Therefore standing does not stop blood from flowing back to the heart.

The increased pressure within the veins of the lower extremities causes them to distend, so that about 500 mL blood is shifted into this part of the circulation. The rise in hydrostatic pressure within the capillaries of the lower extremities increases fluid filtration, causing a progressive loss of plasma volume into the tissues of the legs and feet. The resulting loss of fluid from the central thoracic compartment lowers cardiac output.

These potentially harmful effects are limited by the baroreceptor and cardiopulmonary reflexes, which respond to a fall in the pulse pressure (see Chapter 27). These cause an *increased heart rate* and widespread *vasoconstriction*. This limits the loss of blood from the central thoracic compartment and slightly raises mean arterial blood pressure (MABP) and total peripheral resistance (TPR). The cardiac output falls by about 20%. A local *sympathetic axon reflex* also reduces blood flow to the lower extremities, limiting fluid filtration.

In the upright position, the reduction of intravascular pressures above the heart causes the partial collapse of superficial veins, although the deeper veins remain partly open because their walls are anchored to surrounding tissues. Standing also causes a downward displacement into the spinal canal of the cerebrospinal fluid bathing the central nervous system (CNS), creating a negative pressure inside the rigid cranium that prevents cerebral veins from collapsing. Because cerebral venous pressure is not able to fall as much as arterial pressure, cerebral blood flow decreases by 10–20%.

The skeletal muscle pump

Even during quiet standing, the leg muscles are stimulated by reflexes to contract and relax rhythmically, causing swaying. During contraction, veins within the muscles are squeezed, forcing blood towards the heart, as the venous valves prevent retrograde flow. Upon relaxation, these veins expand, drawing in blood from venules and from superficial veins that communicate with the muscle veins via collaterals (Figure 22). This *skeletal muscle pump* thus 'milks' the veins, driving blood towards the heart to assist venous return. The skeletal muscle pump is greatly potentiated during walking and running, dramatically lowering the venous pressure in the foot to levels as low as 30 mmHg.

The respiratory pump

During inspiration, downward displacement of the diaphragm causes the intrathoracic pressure to fall and the intra-abdominal pressure to rise. This increases the pressure gradient favouring venous return, and vena caval flow rises. An opposite effect occurs during expiration. During straining movements in which there is forced expiration against a closed glottis (e.g. the Valsalva manoeuvre), the rise in intrathoracic pressure severely reduces venous return.

Effect of cardiac contraction

Downward displacement of the ventricles during systole pulls on the atria, expanding them and drawing in blood from the venae cavae and pulmonary veins. When the valves between the atria and ventricles then open during diastole, the blood is drawn in from these veins by the expansion of the ventricles, further aiding venous return. Venous return is therefore driven not only by the upstream pressure, but also (to a smaller extent) by downstream suction.

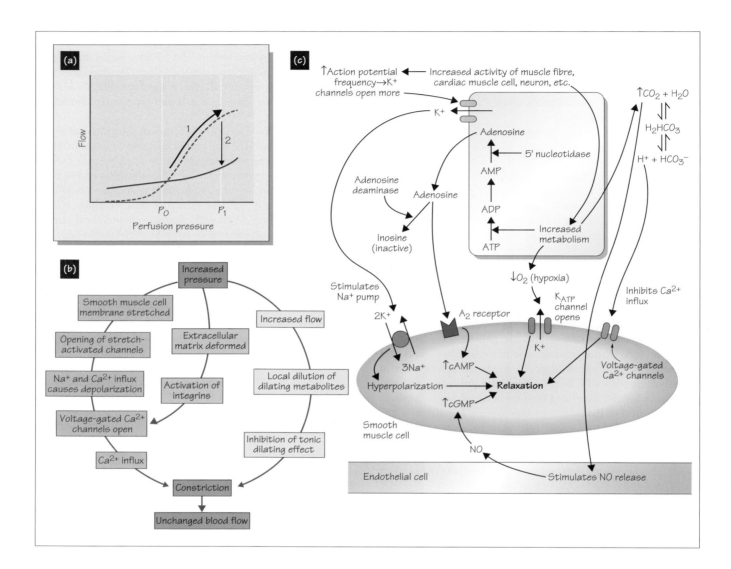

The activity of the sympathetic nervous system provides for centrally coordinated control of vascular tone (see Chapters 27 and 28) and serves to maintain constant arterial blood pressure. However, there are additional mechanisms that regulate vascular tone. Local mechanisms arise either from within the blood vessel itself, or from the surrounding tissue. These local mechanisms function primarily to regulate flow. Regulation tends to be most important in organs that require a constant blood supply, or in which metabolic needs can increase markedly (brain, kidneys, heart, skeletal muscles).

Local mechanisms have two main functions. First, under basal conditions they regulate local vascular resistance to maintain the blood flow in many types of vascular beds at a nearly constant level over a large range of arterial pressures (50–170 mmHg). This tendency to maintain a constant flow during variations in pressure is termed **autoregulation**. Autoregulation prevents major fluctuations in capillary pressure which would lead to uncontrolled movement of fluid into the tissues.

Second, when a tissue requires more blood to meet its metabolic needs, local mechanisms cause dilatation of resistance vessels and upregulate blood flow. This response is referred to as **metabolic vasodilatation**. Autoregulation may persist under these conditions, but is adjusted to maintain flow around the new set point.

Autoregulation

Figure 23a illustrates the phenomenon of autoregulation. When the upstream pressure driving blood through a resistance artery is suddenly increased to P_1 from its starting level P_0, the artery dilates passively and blood flow immediately rises as predicted by Poiseuille's law (arrow 1). However, within a minute the resistance artery responds to the increased pressure by *actively constricting* (arrow 2), thereby bringing blood flow back down towards its initial level (solid line). Similarly, decreases in upstream pressure cause rapid compensatory dilatations to maintain flow. Autoregulation ensures that under basal conditions blood flow remains nearly constant over a wide range of pressures, and is particularly important in the heart, the brain and the kidneys. Two homeostatic negative feedback mechanisms are involved: the **myogenic response** and the effect of **vasodilating metabolites** (Figure 23b).

The myogenic response is probably controlled by sensors in the plasma membrane of vascular smooth muscle cells which react to changes in pressure and/or stretch. There is increasing evidence that **integrins**, membrane-spanning proteins that act as adhesion molecules linking the extracellular matrix with the cytoskeleton (see Chapter 4), may constitute one class of such sensors. Integrins have two subunits (i.e. they are *dimers*), designated α and β, and there are multiple isoforms of each subunit. Recent studies indicate that integrins consisting of $\alpha_5\beta_1$ and $\alpha_v\beta_3$ dimers are necessary for the myogenic response. It is proposed that when pressure increases, changes in the conformation of extracellular matrix proteins occur, and activate the integrins. Integrin activation induces the opening of L-type voltage-gated Ca^{2+} channels, causing Ca^{2+} influx and vasoconstriction. Increased pressure may in addition stimulate **stretch-activated channels**, leading to Na^+ and Ca^{2+} influx, and cell depolarization which is an additional stimulus for opening L-type Ca^{2+} channels. The identities of the stretch-activated channels involved are uncertain, but there is evidence supporting the involvement of two types of **transient receptor potential** (TRP) channels: TRPC6 and TRPM4. The opposite processes (i.e. hyperpolarization, and closing of stretch-activated and voltage-gated Ca^{2+} channels) occur when pressure falls, causing vasodilatation.

Cellular metabolism results in the production of **vasodilating metabolites** or **factors** (Figure 23c) that diffuse into the tissue spaces and affect neighbouring arterioles. If blood flow increases, these substances tend to be washed out of the tissue, leading to an inhibition of vasodilatation that counteracts the rise in blood flow. Conversely, decreased blood flow causes a local accumulation of metabolites, leading to a homeostatic vasodilatation.

Metabolic and reactive hyperaemia

When metabolism in cardiac and skeletal muscle increases during exercise, tissue concentrations of vasodilating metabolites rise markedly. Similarly, focal changes in brain metabolism accompany diverse types of mental activity, causing enhanced local production of metabolites. The increased presence of such factors in the interstitium causes a powerful vasodilatation, termed **metabolic** or **functional hyperaemia**, allowing the rises in blood flow necessary to supply the increased metabolic demand.

An accumulation of vasodilating metabolites also occurs during flow occlusion (e.g. caused by thrombosis). Release of occlusion then results in **reactive hyperaemia**; this is a large increase in blood flow that hastens the re-establishment of cellular energy stores.

This response is transient, persisting until levels of these metabolites fall back to normal.

Metabolic factors

Many factors contribute to metabolic vasodilatation. The most important factors are thought to be **adenosine, K^+ ions** and **hypercapnia** (increased P_{CO_2}). Local **hypoxia** (reduced P_{O_2}) can also relax vascular smooth muscle cells, partly by opening adenosine triphosphate (ATP) sensitive K^+ channels. **Inorganic phosphate, hyperosmolarity** and **lactic acid** may also act as metabolic vasodilators (not shown), although this is less well established.

Adenosine is a potent vasodilator that is released from the heart, skeletal muscles and brain during increased metabolism and hypoxia. It is thought to contribute to metabolic control of blood flow in these organs. Adenosine is produced when adenosine monophosphate (AMP), which accumulates as a result of increased ATP breakdown, is dephosphorylated by the cell membrane enzyme **5′-nucleotidase**. It passes into the extracellular space, dilating neighbouring arterioles before being broken down to inosine by **adenosine deaminase**. It causes vasodilatation by acting on **A_2 receptors** to increase cyclic AMP (cAMP) levels in vascular myocytes. Adenosine also has other actions in the body (e.g. inhibiting conduction in the atrioventricular node), some of which are mediated by **A_1 receptors** (which lower cAMP).

Ischaemia or increased activation of muscles and nerves causes K^+ ions to move out of cells. Resulting increases in the extracellular K^+ concentration (up to 10–15 mmol/L) dilate arterioles, partly by stimulating the Na^+–K^+-ATPase, during functional hyperaemia in skeletal muscle and brain tissue. **Hypercapnia** associated with **acidosis** occurs in brain tissue during stimulation of local metabolism, and also during **cerebral ischaemia** (stroke). These are thought to provide a powerful vasodilating stimulus, both by releasing **nitric oxide** from endothelial cells, and by directly inhibiting Ca^{2+} influx into arteriolar cells.

Other local mechanisms

There are also a number of mechanisms acting locally in selected vascular beds under specific circumstances. For example, during the inflammatory reaction, local infection or trauma causes the release of various **autocoids** (local hormones), including the arteriolar dilators **histamine, prostaglandin E₂, bradykinin** and **platelet activating factor**. These increase local blood flow and increase postcapillary venular permeability, thereby facilitating the access of leucocytes and antibodies to damaged and infected tissues. The generation of **bradykinin** by sweat glands during sweating promotes cutaneous vasodilatation. **Prostaglandin I₂** (PGI₂, prostacyclin) is synthesized and released in the renal cortex under conditions where renal blood flow is reduced by vasoconstrictors. Prostacyclin has a vasodilating action that helps to maintain renal blood flow. Conversely, the release of **serotonin** (5-hydroxytryptamine) and **thromboxane A₂** from platelets during haemostasis causes vasospasm, which helps to reduce bleeding (see Chapter 7).

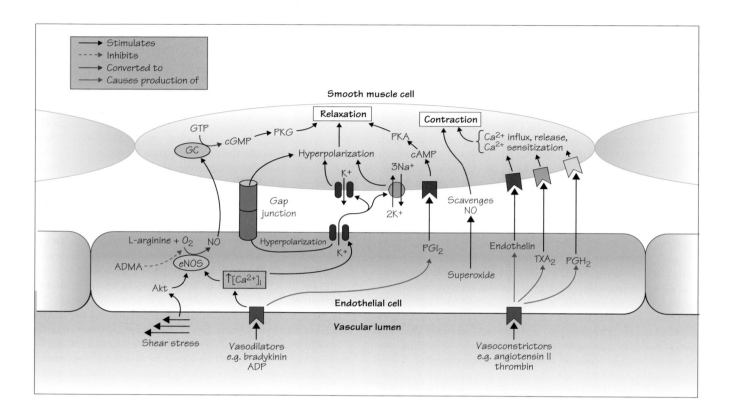

The entire vascular lumen is lined by a monolayer of endothelial cells which are crucial in regulating vascular tone. Endothelial cells can release both constricting and dilating substances when stimulated by blood-borne substances or by shear stress associated with the flow of blood (Figure 24). Important endothelial vasodilators include **nitric oxide** (termed **endothelium-derived relaxing factor** prior to its identification in 1987), **prostacyclin** (PGI_2), and **endothelium-derived hyperpolarizing factor** (EDHF). The major endothelial vasoconstrictors are **endothelin-1, thromboxane A_2** (TXA_2) and **prostaglandin H_2**.

Endothelial cells also have a crucial role in suppressing platelet aggregation and thereby regulating haemostasis (see Chapter 7) and, as the major constituents of the capillary wall, control vascular permeability to many substances (see Chapter 21).

Nitric oxide

Nitric oxide (chemical formula NO) is the major vasodilator released by endothelial cells. NO is synthesized from the amino acid L-arginine and O_2 by nitric oxide synthase (NOS). The most important form of NOS in the cardiovascular system is **endothelial NOS** (eNOS, also NOS-3), which is thought to be responsible for a continual basal production and release of NO by endothelial cells (also by platelets and the heart). eNOS is further activated by a variety of substances that act on their receptors to increase the endothelial cell intracellular Ca^{2+} $[Ca^{2+}]_i$, leading to raised levels of the Ca^{2+} – calmodulin complex which stimulates the enzyme. The

rise in $[Ca^{2+}]_i$ is initiated by Ca^{2+} release from the endoplasmic reticulum, and is subsequently sustained at a lower but still elevated level by Ca^{2+} influx via store-operated Ca^{2+} channels (see Chapter 15). Substances that cause vasodilatation in this way include locally released factors such as bradykinin, adenine, adenosine nucleotides, histamine, serotonin and the neurotransmitter substance P. Acetylcholine has a similar effect, although this probably has little physiological importance in humans.

Shear forces exerted on the endothelium by the flow of blood also activate eNOS, and this contributes to both basal NO release and local regulation of bloodflow. This effect is not caused by a rise in $[Ca^{2+}]_i$, but by cellular pathways activated by shear force-induced deformation of the endothelial cell cytoskeleton. One such pathway involves the sequential activation of the enzymes **phosphatidylinositol 3-kinase (PI3K)** and **Akt**, the latter of which stimulates eNOS via phosphorylation.

Once released from the endothelium, NO diffuses through the vascular wall and into the smooth muscle cells, where it activates the cytosolic enzyme **guanylyl cyclase**. This increases levels of cellular cyclic GMP, which causes relaxation as described in Chapter 15.

NO is a free radical (i.e. it contains an unpaired electron) and is therefore very reactive. In particular, upon its release NO reacts very rapidly with **superoxide**, another free radical which is continually being produced by a variety of enzymes (including eNOS) to form **peroxynitrite**, a substance that does not cause vasodilatation,

The Cardiovascular System at a Glance, Fourth Edition. Philip I. Aaronson, Jeremy P.T. Ward, and Michelle J. Connolly.

and which in excess may damage cells. Because any given molecule of NO therefore survives for only a few seconds, the effects of NO are exerted locally and require its continued production.

Neuronal NOS (nNOS, also NOS-1) is expressed by multiple types of cells, including autonomic and sensory nerves, vascular smooth muscle and skeletal muscle fibres. Local release of NO by nNOS in the macula densa is important in regulating renal blood flow, and recent findings indicate that continual NO production by nNOS in arteries and/or skeletal muscle probably acts as a tonic vasodilating influence on arteries and arterioles throughout the body.

Inducible NOS (iNOS, also NOS-2) is expressed in macrophages, lymphocytes, vascular smooth muscle and other types of cells during inflammation. iNOS is capable of producing much greater amounts of NO and probably aids destruction of foreign organisms by the immune system. An overproduction of NO by iNOS in septic shock is thought to contribute to the severe hypotension characterizing this condition.

The formation of NO is competitively antagonized by drugs such as the non-selective NOS inhibitor L-nitro arginine methyl ester (L-NAME) and the selective nNOS blocker S-methyl-L-thiocitrulline (SMTC). These are useful experimental tools for evaluating the roles of NO *in vitro* and *in vivo*. Remarkably, an *endogenous* competitive inhibitor of eNOS called **ADMA** (asymmetric dimethyl arginine) is normally present in the plasma at a concentration of $\sim 1\,\mu mol/L$, and is formed by **protein arginine methyltransferases**, enzymes in the nucleus that attach methyl groups to arginine residues in proteins. Subsequent protein hydrolysis then releases ADMA. ADMA is metabolized by the ubiquitous enzyme **dimethylarginine dimethylaminohydrolase**, and is also excreted by the kidneys. Elevated plasma levels of ADMA are a cardiovascular risk factor, and occur in diabetes mellitus, hyperhomocysteinaemia and pre-eclampsia.

Other endothelium-derived relaxing mechanisms

Many of the factors that evoke endothelial NO production also stimulate the endothelial release of prostacyclin and EDHF. Prostacyclin promotes vasodilatation by increasing smooth muscle cell cyclic AMP levels, but its most important role is in limiting platelet attachment and aggregation.

EDHF was originally defined as a substance or substances released from the endothelium that cause(s) smooth muscle hyperpolarization (and therefore relaxation, see Chapter 15) by opening K$^+$ channels and/or stimulating the activity of the Na$^+$ pump, and is particularly important in causing dilatation of arterioles, where its influence may exceed that of NO. The EDHF response is now thought to occur because the rises in endothelial cell [Ca^{2+}] that trigger NO and PGI$_2$ synthesis also open Ca^{2+} activated K$^+$ channels in these cells. This causes a hyperpolarization of the endothelial cells which is transmitted directly to the surrounding smooth muscle cells through **myoendothelial gap junctions** which connect these two types of cells and allow current to flow between them. The opening of endothelial cell K$^+$ channels also raises the extracellular [K$^+$] around the smooth muscle cells that are adjacent to the endothelium, and this further promotes smooth muscle cell hyperpolarization by activating both the Na$^+$ pump and the **inward recti-**

fier (K$_{IR}$), a type of K$^+$ channel that has the unusual property of allowing a greater efflux of K$^+$ when the extracellular [K$^+$] increases. **Hydrogen peroxide** and **epoxyeicosatrienoic acids**, which are produced from arachidonic acid by the enzyme cytochrome P450, have also been proposed as EDHFs. However, recent work indicates that they both act in an autocrine manner on endothelial cells to promote rises in [Ca^{2+}]$_i$ and therefore K$^+$ efflux, thereby enhancing rather than causing the EDHF response.

Endothelium-derived constricting factors

Endothelin-1 is a 21 amino acid peptide that is released from the endothelium by many vasoconstrictors, including angiotensin, vasopressin, thrombin and adrenaline. Endothelin is a potent vasoconstricting agent, particularly in veins and arterioles, and stimulates two subtypes of receptor on vascular smooth muscle cells, designated ET$_A$ and ET$_B$ Endothelin causes vasoconstriction via G-protein-linked mechanisms similar to those activated by noradrenaline. The infusion of endothelin receptor antagonists into humans causes a sustained fall in total peripheral resistance, implying that ongoing endothelin release contributes to maintaining the blood pressure.

Endothelial cells can also release other vasoconstricting substances, including **prostanoids** (thromboxane A$_2$ and prostaglandin H$_2$), and superoxide anions which may enhance constriction by breaking down NO. In addition, **angiotensin-converting enzyme** (ACE) present on the surface of endothelial cells converts is responsible for both the production of the vasoconstrictor angiotensin II (see Chapters 29 and 35) and the breakdown of the potent vasodilator bradykinin.

Endothelium in cardiovascular disease

Many diseases that disturb vascular function are associated with abnormalities of the endothelium. Dysfunction of the endothelium is thought to contribute to the early stages of **atherosclerosis**, while damage to the endothelium is a crucial factor leading to thrombus formation in the advanced atherosclerotic lesion (see Chapter 37). Plasma from patients with **diabetes mellitus** contains abnormally high levels of biochemical markers indicative of endothelial damage, and there is evidence, both in animal models of insulin-dependent diabetes and in patients with this disorder, for blunted endothelium-dependent relaxation. This deficit in endothelial function is thought to contribute to the increased risks of atherosclerosis, neuropathy and hypertension that are associated with diabetes. The mechanisms leading to diabetes-associated endothelial dysfunction remain incompletely defined, but may include damage by raised levels of glucose and/or oxidized low density lipoproteins.

Endothelial dysfunction may also be important in causing **pre-eclampsia**, a disorder of pregnancy characterized by hypertension and increased blood clotting, which is the leading cause of maternal mortality. The endothelium is thought to have an important role in causing the fall in maternal blood pressure that normally occurs during pregnancy. However, this protective function may be disrupted in patients with pre-eclampsia, possibly because of the release of substances from the placenta that damage the endothelial cells.

The coronary, cutaneous and cerebral circulations

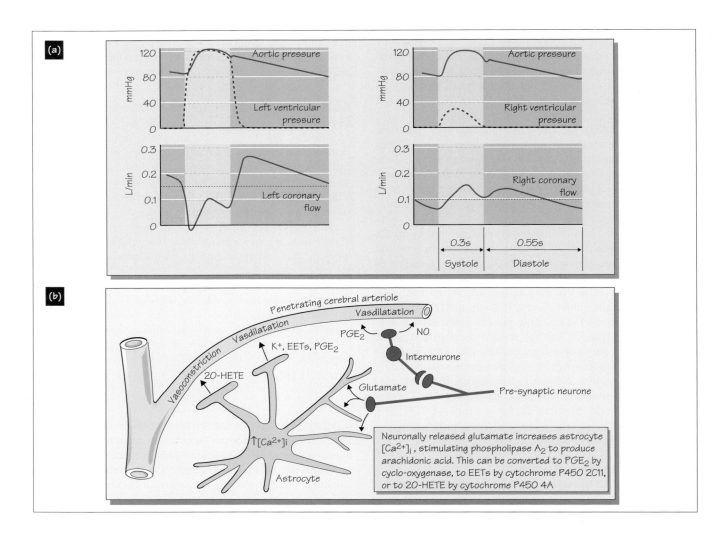

The vascular beds supplying the different organs of the body are structurally and functionally specialized, allowing an optimal matching of blood flow with their individual requirements.

Coronary circulation

The anatomy of the coronary circulation is described in Chapter 2.

The *high capillary density* of the myocardium (~1 capillary per muscle cell) allows it to extract an unusually large fraction (about 70%) of the oxygen from its blood supply. The resting blood flow to the heart is relatively high, and moreover increases approximately fivefold during strenuous exercise.

Figure 25a shows left and right coronary blood flow during the cardiac cycle at a resting heart rate (HR) of 70 beats/min. During systole, the branches of the left coronary artery that penetrate the myocardial wall to supply the subendocardium of the left ventricle are strongly compressed by the high pressure within the ventricle and its wall. Left coronary blood flow is therefore almost abol-

ished during systole, so that 85% of flow occurs during diastole. Conversely, right coronary arterial flow rate is highest during systole, because the aortic pressure driving flow increases more during systole (from 80 to 120 mmHg) than the right ventricular pressure which opposes flow (from 0 to 25 mmHg).

With a HR of 70 beats/min, systole and diastole last 0.3 and 0.55 s, respectively. As the HR increases during exercise or excitement, however, the duration of diastole shortens more than that of systole. At 200 beats/min, for example, systole and diastole both last for 0.15 s. In order to cope with the greatly increased oxygen demand of the heart, which occurs simultaneously with a marked reduction in the time available for left coronary perfusion, the coronary arteries/arterioles dilate dramatically to allow for a pronounced rise in blood flow. The mechanism of this **exercise hyperaemia** in humans is unknown. However, in the porcine coronary circulation, which seems to be regulated in a manner similar to that of humans, coronary exercise hyperaemia is probably caused by reduction of endothelin release from the coronary endothelium,

The Cardiovascular System at a Glance, Fourth Edition. Philip I. Aaronson, Jeremy P.T. Ward, and Michelle J. Connolly.

plus a sympathetically mediated β-receptor activation of coronary artery smooth muscle which results in a rise in cellular cyclic AMP (cAMP) and the opening of BK_{Ca} channels.

Cutaneous circulation

Apart from supplying the relatively modest metabolic requirements of the skin, the main function of the cutaneous vasculature is **thermoregulation**, the maintenance of a constant body temperature. Vascular tone in the skin is regulated by both neural reflexes and local cutaneous mechanisms that respond to temperature. Temperature increases cause cutaneous vasodilatation, allowing more blood to flow to the skin and radiate its heat to the environment to promote body cooling; decreases in temperature have the opposite effect.

Neural control of cutaneous vascular tone is exerted by two types of sympathetic nerves. A **sympathetic vasoconstrictor system** is tonically active under thermoneutral conditions. A fall in body temperature, sensed by peripheral and hypothalamic thermoreceptors, further activates this system, causing the release of noradrenaline which acts through α_1 and α_2 receptors to trigger cutaneous vasoconstriction. This minimizes the loss of body heat by producing a pronounced decrease in cutaneous blood flow, which can fall to one-tenth of its thermoneutral level of 10–20 mL/min/100 g. With increased temperatures, these nerves are inhibited and cutaneous blood vessels open, bringing blood to the skin to increase sweating and heat loss. These nerves innervate both **glabrous** skin (the skin of the *hands*, *feet*, *lips*, *nose* and *ears*) and non-glabrous skin. In glabrous skin, they control the constriction of **arteriovenous anastomoses** (AVAs) which are coiled, thick-walled thoroughfare blood vessels that connect arterioles and veins directly, bypassing the capillaries. When open, AVAs allow a high volume blood flow into a cutaneous venous plexus (network) from which heat can be radiated to the environment. Non-glabrous skin lacks AVAs.

A **sympathetic vasodilator system**, which innervates non-glabrous skin only, is inactive under thermoneutral or cool conditions. It becomes active when the core body temperature rises, and is responsible for ~90% of the very large (up to 30-fold) increase in the flow of blood to the skin that can occur at high temperatures. Although these are cholinergic nerves, vasodilatation is probably caused by putative co-transmitters such as NO and substance P rather than acetylcholine.

Local skin temperature also affects cutaneous blood vessels. Local heating causes cutaneous vasodilatation which is thought to depend on NO and also a local reflex involving sensory nerves. Local cooling induces cutaneous vasoconstriction. This is probably due to inhibition of NO release or effect, as well as an increased action of noradrenaline on vascular smooth muscle cell α_{2C} receptors, more of which are inserted into the cell membrane as the temperature drops. However, prolonged cold causes a paradoxical vasodilatation. Cutaneous vessels are also constricted by the baroreceptor reflex, helping to increase total peripheral resistance (TPR) and shift blood to the vital organs during haemorrhage or shock. This involvement of the cutaneous vasculature in the baroreceptor reflex is particularly important at elevated body temperatures, when >50% of the cardiac output may be directed to the skin.

Cerebral circulation

The brain receives about 15% of cardiac output. The **basilar** and **internal carotid arteries** entering the cranium join to form an arterial ring, the **circle of Willis**, from which arise the **anterior**, **middle** and **posterior cerebral arteries** which supply the cranium. This arrangement helps to defend the cerebral blood supply, which if occluded causes immediate unconsciousness and irreversible tissue damage within minutes.

The brain, especially the neuronal grey matter, has a very high capillary density (~3000–4000 capillaries/mm³) and blood flow. Coupled with a large (~35%) fractional O_2 extraction, this allows it to sustain the high rate of oxidative metabolism it requires to function. The arteriolar myogenic response is well developed, allowing cerebral blood flow to be maintained constant at arterial pressures between about 50 and 170 mmHg. **CO₂** concentrations in the surrounding brain are particularly important in causing vasodilatation (see Chapter 23). The effect of CO_2 is in part caused by NO release from endothelial cells. Hyperventilation, which reduces arterial CO_2, can cause a marked cerebral vasoconstriction and temporary unconsciousness. Sympathetic regulation of the blood flow to the brain exists, but is probably of minor importance.

Increased neuronal activity dilates local arterioles within seconds through several mechanisms (Figure 25b). Some neurones release transmitters such as NO, vasoactive intestinal peptide or prostaglandin E_2 (PGE_2), which are vasodilators. Neuronal activity also regulates intracerebral arterioles indirectly via effects on **astrocytes**. These are glial cells that have 'endfeet' that are in close contact with adjacent arterioles (in fact arterioles within the brain are almost completely encased in astrocytic endfeet). Astrocytes also have multitudinous projections that surround and monitor the activity of >100 000 neuronal synapses and respond to increased activity in their synaptic 'domain' by raising their intracellular Ca^{2+} concentration. This is thought to cause them to release substances such as K^+, PGE_2 and epoxyeicosatrienoic acids (EETs) from their endfeet onto the arterioles, causing them to dilate. They may also be able to elicit vasoconstriction by releasing 20-hydroxyeicosatetraenoic acid (20-HETE). Astrocytes are coupled to each other electrically by gap junctions, forming a network that may act to spread the vasodilating 'message' upsteam so that the larger arteries feeding regions of increased neuronal activity also dilate.

The brain and spinal cord float in the **cerebrospinal fluid** (CSF), which is contained within the rigid cranium and the spinal canal. Because the cranium is rigid and its contents are incompressible, the volume of blood within the brain remains roughly constant, and increases in arterial inflow are compensated for by decreases in venous volume. By increasing the tissue mass, brain tumours increase the intracerebral pressure and reduce cerebral blood flow. Increased intracerebral pressure is partially compensated for by the **Cushing reflex**, a characteristic rise in arterial pressure associated with a reflex bradycardia.

The pulmonary, skeletal muscle and fetal circulations

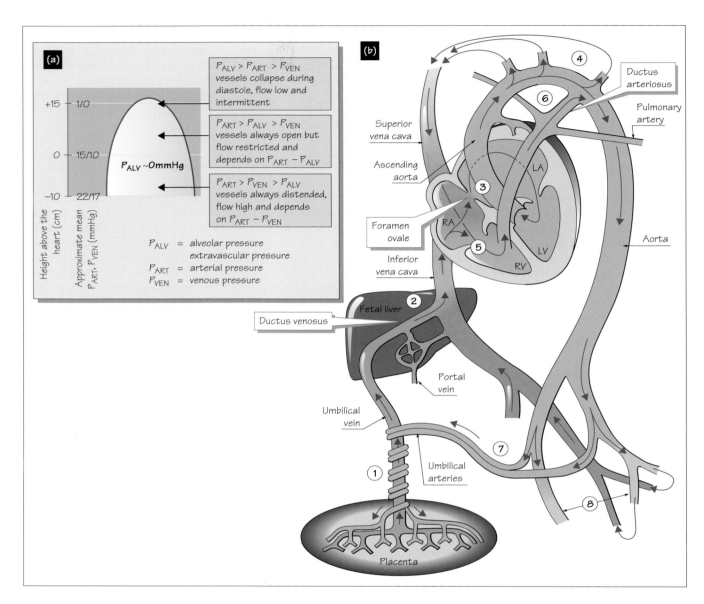

(a)

$P_{ALV} > P_{ART} > P_{VEN}$ vessels collapse during diastole, flow low and intermittent

$P_{ART} > P_{ALV} > P_{VEN}$ vessels always open but flow restricted and depends on $P_{ART} - P_{ALV}$

$P_{ART} > P_{VEN} > P_{ALV}$ vessels always distended, flow high and depends on $P_{ART} - P_{VEN}$

+15   1/0

0   15/10

−10   22/17

$P_{ALV} \sim 0\,mmHg$

Height above the heart (cm)

Approximate mean P_{ART}, P_{VEN} (mmHg)

P_{ALV} = alveolar pressure extravascular pressure
P_{ART} = arterial pressure
P_{VEN} = venous pressure

(b)

Ductus arteriosus

Pulmonary artery

Superior vena cava

Ascending aorta

Foramen ovale

Inferior vena cava

Ductus venosus

Fetal liver

Portal vein

Umbilical vein

Umbilical arteries

Placenta

Aorta

RA, LA, RV, LV

The pulmonary circulation

As described in Chapter 1, the **pulmonary circulation** receives the entire output of the right ventricle. Its high-density capillary network surrounds the lung alveoli, allowing the O_2-poor blood from the pulmonary arteries to exchange CO_2 for O_2. The pulmonary veins return highly oxygenated blood to the left atrium. The pulmonary circulation contains about 800 mL of blood in recumbent subjects, falling to about 450 mL during quiet standing.

Mean pulmonary arterial pressure is ~15 mmHg, and left atrial pressure is ~5 mmHg. The right ventricle is able to drive its entire output through the pulmonary circulation utilizing a pressure head of only 10 mmHg because the resistance of the pulmonary circulation is only 10–15% that of the systemic circulation. This arises because the vessels of the pulmonary microcirculation are short and of relatively wide bore, with little resting tone. They are also very

numerous, so that their total cross-section is similar to that of the systemic circulation. The walls of both arteries and veins are thin and distensible, and contain comparatively little smooth muscle.

The low pressure within the pulmonary circulation means that regional perfusion of the lungs in the upright position is greatly affected by gravity (Figure 26a). The extravascular pressure throughout the lungs is similar to the alveolar pressure (~0 mmHg). However, the intravascular pressure is low in the lung apices, which are above the heart, and high in the lung bases, which are below the heart. Pulmonary vessels in the lung apices therefore collapse during diastole, causing intermittent flow. Conversely, vessels in the bases of the lungs are perfused throughout the cardiac cycle, and are distended. A small increase in pulmonary arterial pressure during exercise is sufficient to open up apical capillaries, allowing more O_2 uptake by the blood.

The Cardiovascular System at a Glance, Fourth Edition. Philip I. Aaronson, Jeremy P.T. Ward, and Michelle J. Connolly.

The low hydrostatic pressure in pulmonary capillaries (mean of 7–10 mmHg) does not lead to net fluid resorption, because it is balanced by a low extravascular hydrostatic pressure and an unusually high interstitial plasma protein oncotic pressure (~18 mmHg). The lung capillaries therefore produce a small net flow of lymph, which is drained by an extensive pulmonary lymphatic network. During left ventricular failure or mitral stenosis, however, the increased left atrial pressure backs up into the pulmonary circulation, increasing fluid filtration and leading to **pulmonary oedema**.

Neither the sympathetic nervous system nor myogenic/metabolic autoregulation have much of a role in regulating pulmonary vascular resistance or flow. However, the pulmonary vasculature is well supplied with sympathetic nerves. When stimulated, these decrease the compliance of the vessels, limiting the pulmonary blood volume so that more blood is available to the systemic circulation.

The most important mechanism regulating pulmonary vascular tone is **hypoxic pulmonary vasoconstriction** (HPV), a process by which pulmonary vessels *constrict* in response to alveolar **hypoxia**. This unique mechanism (systemic vessels typically *dilate* to hypoxia) diverts blood away from poorly ventilated regions of the lungs, thereby maximizing the **ventilation – perfusion ratio**. HPV is probably caused mainly by hypoxia-induced release of Ca^{2+} from the sarcoplasmic reticulum within the smooth muscle cells of the pulmonary vasculature.

The skeletal muscle circulation

The skeletal muscles comprise about 50% of body weight, and at rest receive 15–20% of cardiac output. At rest, skeletal muscle arterioles have a high basal tone as a result of tonic sympathetic vasoconstriction. At any one time, most muscle capillaries are not perfused, due to intermittent constriction of precapillary sphincters (vasomotion).

Because the muscles form such a large tissue mass, their arterioles make a major contribution to total peripheral resistance (TPR). Sympathetically mediated alterations in their arteriolar tone therefore have a crucial role in regulating TPR and blood pressure during operation of the baroreceptor reflex. The muscles thus serve as a '*pressure valve*' that can be closed to increase blood pressure and opened to lower it.

With *rhythmic* exercise, compression of blood vessels during the contraction phase causes the blood flow to become intermittent. However, increased muscle metabolism causes the generation of *vasodilating factors*; these factors cause an enormous increase in blood flow during the relaxation phase, especially to the white or phasic fibres involved in movement. With maximal exercise, the skeletal muscles receive 80–90% of cardiac output. Vasodilating factors include **K^+ ions**, **CO_2** and **hyperosmolarity**. In working muscle their effects completely *override* sympathetic vasoconstriction, while arterioles in non-working muscle remain sympathetically constricted so that their blood flow does not increase.

Sustained compression of blood vessels during *static* (isometric) muscle contractions causes an occlusion of flow that rapidly results in muscle fatigue.

The fetal circulation

A diagram of the fetal circulation is shown in Figure 26b. The fetus receives O_2 and nutrients from, and discharges CO_2 and metabolic waste products into, the maternal circulation. This exchange occurs in the **placenta**, a thick spongy pancake-shaped structure lying between the fetus and the uterine wall. The placenta is composed of a space containing maternal blood, which is packed with **fetal villi**, branching tree-like structures containing fetal arteries, capillaries and veins. They receive the fetal blood from branches of the two **umbilical arteries**, and drain back into the fetus via the **umbilical vein**. Gas and nutrient exchange occurs between the fetal capillaries in the villi and the maternal blood surrounding and bathing the villi.

The fetal circulation differs from that of adults in that *the right and left ventricles pump the blood in parallel rather than in series*. This arrangement allows the heart and head to receive more highly oxygenated blood, and is made possible by three structural *shunts* unique to the fetus: the **ductus venosus**, the **foramen ovale** and the **ductus arteriosus** (highlighted in Figure 26b).

Blood leaving the placenta (**1**) via the umbilical vein is 80% saturated with O_2. About half of this flows into the fetal liver. The rest is diverted into the inferior vena cava via the **ductus venosus** (**2**), mixing with poorly oxygenated venous blood returning from the fetus' lower body. When the resulting relatively oxygen-rich mixture (about 67% saturated) enters the right atrium, most of it does not pass into the right ventricle as it would in the adult, but is directed into the left atrium via the **foramen ovale**, an opening between the fetal atria (**3**). Blood then flows into the left ventricle, and is pumped into the ascending aorta, from which it perfuses the head, the coronary circulation and the arms (**4**). Venous blood from these areas re-enters the heart via the superior vena cava. This blood, now about 35% saturated with O_2, mixes with the fraction of blood from the inferior vena cava not entering the foramen ovale (**5**), and flows into the right ventricle, which pumps it into the pulmonary artery. Instead of then entering the lungs, as it would in the adult, about 90% of the blood leaving the right ventricle is diverted into the descending aorta through the **ductus arteriosus** (**6**). This occurs because pressure in the pulmonary circulation is higher than that in the systemic circulation, as a result of pulmonary vasoconstriction and the collapsed state of the lungs. About 60% of blood entering the descending aorta then flows back to the placenta for oxygenation (**7**). The rest, now 58% saturated with O_2, supplies the fetus' trunk and legs (**8**).

Circulatory changes at birth

Two events at birth quickly cause the fetal circulation to assume a quasi-adult pattern. First, the pulmonary vascular pressure falls well below the systemic pressure because of the initiation of breathing and the resulting pulmonary vasodilatation. Together with constriction of the ductus arteriosus caused by increased blood O_2 levels, this reversal of the pulmonary – systemic pressure gradient, which is aided by the loss of the low-resistance placental circulation, abolishes the blood flow from the pulmonary artery into the aorta within 30 min after delivery.

Second, tying off the umbilical cord stops venous return from the placenta, abruptly lowering inferior vena caval pressure. Together with the fall in pulmonary resistance, this lowers right atrial pressure, causing within hours functional closure of the foramen ovale. The ductus venosus also closes with the abolition of venous return from the placenta.

Although these fetal circulatory shunts are *functionally* closed soon after birth, complete *structural* closure only occurs after several months. In 20% of adults, the structural closure of the foramen ovale remains incomplete, although this is of no haemodynamic consequence.

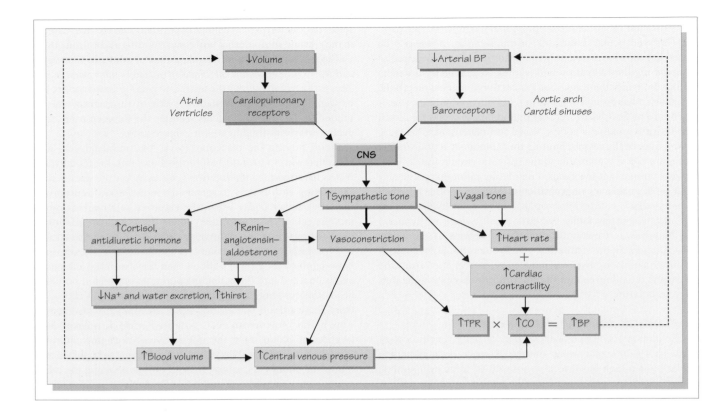

The cardiovascular system is centrally regulated by **autonomic reflexes**. These work with local mechanisms (see Chapter 23) and the **renin – angiotension – aldosterone** and **antidiuretic hormone** systems (see Chapter 29) to minimize fluctuations in the mean arterial blood pressure (MABP) and volume, and to maintain adequate cerebral and coronary perfusion. **Intrinsic** reflexes, including the **baroreceptor**, **cardiopulmonary** and **chemoreceptor** reflexes, respond to stimuli originating within the cardiovascular system. Less important **extrinsic** reflexes mediate the cardiovascular response to stimuli originating elsewhere (e.g. pain, temperature changes). Figure 27 illustrates the responses of the baroreceptor and cardiopulmonary reflexes to reduced blood pressure and volume, as would occur, for example, during haemorrhage.

Cardiovascular reflexes involve three components:

1 Afferent nerves ('receptors') sense a change in the state of the system, and communicate this to the brain, which

2 Processes this information and implements an appropriate response, by

3 Altering the activity of efferent nerves controlling cardiac, vascular and renal function, thereby causing homeostatic responses that reverse the change in state.

Intrinsic cardiovascular reflexes
The baroreceptor reflex
This reflex acts rapidly to minimize moment-to-moment fluctuations in the MABP. **Baroreceptors** are afferent (sensory) nerve endings in the walls of the **carotid sinuses** (thin-walled dilatations at the origins of the internal carotid arteries) and the **aortic arch**. These **mechanoreceptors** sense alterations in wall stretch caused by pressure changes, and respond by modifying the frequency at which they fire action potentials. Pressure elevations increase impulse frequency; pressure decreases have the opposite effect.

When MABP decreases, the fall in baroreceptor impulse frequency causes the brain to *reduce* the firing of vagal efferents supplying the sinoatrial node, thus causing tachycardia. Simultaneously, the activity of sympathetic nerves innervating the heart and most blood vessels is *increased*, causing increased cardiac contractility and constriction of arteries and veins. Stimulation of renal sympathetic nerves increases renin release, and consequently angiotensin II production and aldosterone secretion (see Chapter 29). The resulting tachycardia, vasoconstriction and fluid retention act together to raise MABP. Opposite effects occur when arterial blood pressure rises.

There are two types of baroreceptors. **A fibres** have large, myelinated axons and are activated over lower levels of pressure. **C fibres** have small, unmyelinated axons and respond over higher levels of pressure. Together, these provide an input to the brain which is most sensitive to pressure changes between 80 and 150 mmHg. The brain is able to reset the baroreflex to allow increases in MABP to occur (e.g. during exercise and the defence reaction). Ageing, hypertension and atherosclerosis decrease arterial wall compliance, reducing baroreceptor reflex sensitivity.

The Cardiovascular System at a Glance, Fourth Edition. Philip I. Aaronson, Jeremy P.T. Ward, and Michelle J. Connolly.

The baroreceptors quickly show partial *adaptation* to new pressure levels. Therefore alterations in frequency are greatest while pressure is changing, and tend to moderate when a new steady-state pressure level is established. If unable to prevent a change in MABP, the reflex will within several hours become *reset* to maintain pressure around the new level. This finding, together with studies by Cowley and coworkers in the 1970s showing that destroying baroreceptor function increased the variability of MABP but had little effect on its average value measured over a long time, led to general acceptance of the idea that baroreceptors have no role in long-term regulation of MABP. However, recent evidence that baroreceptor resetting is incomplete and that electrical stimulation of baroreceptors causes reductions in MABP which are sustained over many days has led some experts to re-evaluate this issue.

Cardiopulmonary reflexes

Diverse intrinsic cardiovascular reflexes originate in the heart and lungs. Cutting the vagal afferent fibres mediating these **cardiopulmonary reflexes** causes an increased heart rate and vasoconstriction, especially in muscle, renal and mesenteric vascular beds. Cardiopulmonary reflexes are therefore thought to exert a *net tonic depression of the heart rate and vascular tone*. Receptors for these reflexes are located mainly in *low-pressure regions* of the cardiovascular system, and are well placed to sense the *blood volume* in the central thoracic compartment. These reflexes are thought to be particularly important in controlling blood volume, as well as vascular tone, and act together with the baroreceptors to stabilize the MABP. However, these reflexes have been studied mainly in animals, and their specific individual roles in humans are incompletely understood.

Specific components of the cardiopulmonary reflexes include the following.

1 Atrial mechanoreceptors with non-myelinated vagal afferents which respond to increased atrial volume/pressure by causing bradycardia and vasodilatation.

2 Mechanoreceptors in the left ventricle and coronary arteries with mainly non-myelinated vagal afferents which respond to increased ventricular diastolic pressure and afterload by causing a vasodilatation.

3 Ventricular chemoreceptors which are stimulated by substances such as bradykinin and prostaglandins released during cardiac ischaemia. These receptors activate the **coronary chemoreflex**. This response, also termed the **Bezold – Jarisch effect**, occurs after the intravenous injection of many drugs, and involves marked bradycardia and widespread vasodilatation.

4 Pulmonary mechanoreceptors, which when activated by marked lung inflation, especially if oedema is present, cause tachycardia and vasodilatation.

5 Mechanoreceptors with myelinated vagal afferents, located mainly at the juncture of the atria and great veins, which respond to increased atrial volume and pressure by causing a sympathetically mediated tachycardia (**Bainbridge reflex**). This reflex also helps to control blood volume; its activation decreases the secretion of **antidiuretic hormone** (vasopressin), **cortisol** and **renin**, causing a diuresis. Although powerful in dogs, this reflex has been difficult to demonstrate in humans.

Chemoreceptor reflexes

Chemoreceptors activated by **hypoxia**, **hypocapnia** and **acidosis** are located in the aortic and carotid bodies. These are stimulated during asphyxia, hypoxia and severe hypotension. The resulting **chemoreceptor reflex** is mainly involved in stimulating breathing, but also has cardiovascular effects. These include sympathetic constriction of (mainly skeletal muscle) arterioles, splanchnic venoconstriction and a tachycardia resulting indirectly from the increased lung inflation. This reflex is important in maintaining blood flow to the brain at arterial pressures too low to affect baroreceptor activity.

The CNS ischaemic response

Brainstem hypoxia stimulates a powerful generalized peripheral vasoconstriction. This response develops during severe hypotension, helping to maintain the flow of blood to the brain during shock. It also causes the **Cushing reflex**, in which vasoconstriction and hypertension develop when increased cerebrospinal fluid pressure (e.g. due to a brain tumour) produces brainstem hypoxia.

Extrinsic reflexes

Stimuli that are external to the cardiovascular system also exert effects on the heart and vasculature via extrinsic reflexes. Moderate pain causes tachycardia and increases MABP; however, severe pain has the opposite effects. Cold causes cutaneous and coronary vasoconstriction, possibly precipitating angina in susceptible individuals.

Central regulation of cardiovascular reflexes

The afferent nerves carrying impulses from cardiovascular receptors terminate in the **nucleus tractus solitarius** (NTS) of the medulla. Neurones from the NTS project to areas of the brainstem that control both parasympathetic and sympathetic outflow, influencing their level of activation. The **nucleus ambiguus** and **dorsal motor nucleus** contain the cell bodies of the preganglionic vagal parasympathetic neurones, which slow the heart when the cardiovascular receptors report an increased blood pressure to the NTS. Neurones from the NTS also project to areas of **ventrolateral medulla**; from these descend bulbospinal fibres which influence the firing of the sympathetic preganglionic neurons in the intermediolateral (IML) columns of the spinal cord.

These neural circuits are capable of mediating the basic cardiovascular reflexes. However, the NTS, the other brainstem centres and the IML neurones receive descending inputs from the hypothalamus, which in turn is influenced by impulses from the limbic system of the cerebral cortex. Input from these higher centres modifies the activity of the brainstem centres, allowing the generation of integrated responses in which the functions of the cardiovascular system and other organs are coordinated in such a way that the appropriate responses to changing conditions can be orchestrated.

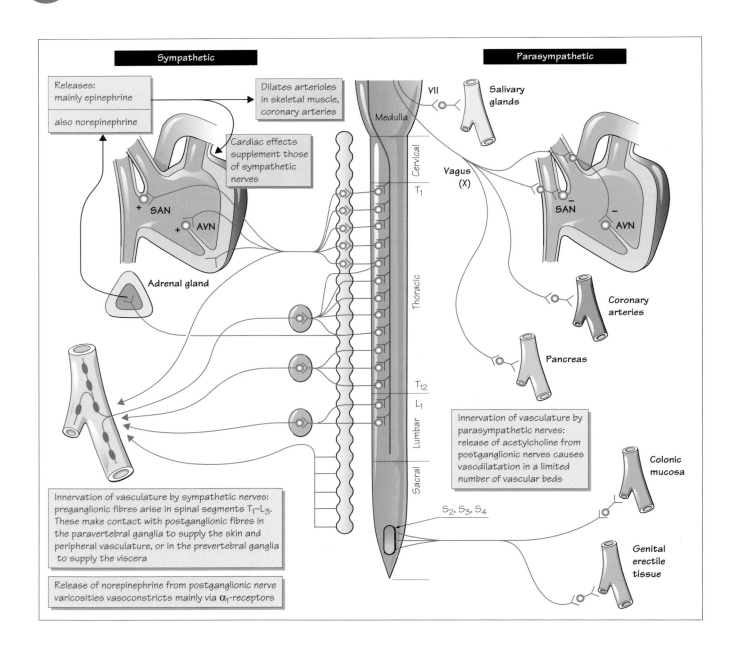

Sympathetic

Releases:
mainly epinephrine

also norepinephrine

Dilates arterioles
in skeletal muscle,
coronary arteries

Cardiac effects
supplement those
of sympathetic
nerves

Medulla

Cervical

T_1

Thoracic

T_{12}

L_1

Lumbar

Sacral

+ SAN

+ AVN

Adrenal gland

Innervation of vasculature by sympathetic nerves:
preganglionic fibres arise in spinal segments T_1–L_3.
These make contact with postganglionic fibres in
the paravertebral ganglia to supply the skin and
peripheral vasculature, or in the prevertebral ganglia
to supply the viscera

Release of norepinephrine from postganglionic nerve
varicosities vasoconstricts mainly via α_1-receptors

Parasympathetic

VII

Salivary
glands

Vagus
(X)

SAN

AVN

Coronary
arteries

Pancreas

Innervation of vasculature by
parasympathetic nerves:
release of acetylcholine from
postganglionic nerves causes
vasodilatation in a limited
number of vascular beds

S_2, S_3, S_4

Colonic
mucosa

Genital
erectile
tissue

The Cardiovascular System at a Glance, Fourth Edition. Philip I. Aaronson, Jeremy P.T. Ward, and Michelle J. Connolly.

The **autonomic nervous system** (ANS) comprises a *system of efferent nerves* that regulate the involuntary functioning of most organs, including the heart and vasculature. The cardiovascular effects of the ANS are deployed for two purposes.

First, the ANS provides the effector arm of the cardiovascular *reflexes*, which respond mainly to activation of receptors in the cardiovascular system (see Chapter 27). They are designed to maintain an *appropriate blood pressure*, and have a crucial role in homeostatic adjustments to *postural changes* (see Chapter 22), *haemorrhage* (see Chapter 31) and *changes in blood gases*. The autonomic circulation is able to override local vascular control mechanisms in order to serve the needs of the body as a whole.

Second, ANS function is also regulated by signals initiated within the brain as it reacts to *environmental stimuli* or *emotional stress*. The brain can selectively modify or override the cardiovascular reflexes, producing specific patterns of cardiovascular adjustments, which are sometimes coupled with behavioural responses. Complex responses of this type are involved in *exercise* (see Chapter 30), *thermoregulation* (see Chapter 25), the *'fight or flight' (defence) response* and *'playing dead'*.

The ANS is divided into **sympathetic** and **parasympathetic** branches. The nervous pathways of both branches of the ANS consist of two sets of neurones arranged in series. **Preganglionic neurones** originate in the central nervous system and terminate in peripheral **ganglia**, where they synapse with **postganglionic neurones** innervating the target organs.

The sympathetic system

Sympathetic preganglionic neurones originate in the **intermediolateral** (IML) columns of the spinal cord. These neurones exit the spinal cord through ventral roots of segments T_1–L_2, and synapse with the postganglionic fibres in either **paravertebral** or **prevertebral** ganglia. The paravertebral ganglia are arranged in two sympathetic chains, one of which is shown in Figure 28. These are located on either side of the spinal cord, and usually contain 22 or 23 ganglia. The prevertebral ganglia, shown to the left of the sympathetic chain, are diffuse structures that form part of the visceral autonomic plexuses of the abdomen and pelvis. The ganglionic neurotransmitter is **acetylcholine**, and it activates postganglionic **nicotinic cholinergic** receptors.

The postganglionic fibres terminate in the effector organs, where they release **noradrenaline**. Preganglionic sympathetic fibres also control the **adrenal medulla**, which releases **adrenaline** and noradrenaline into the blood. Under physiological conditions, the effect of neuronal noradrenaline release is more important than that of adrenaline and noradrenaline released by the adrenal medulla.

Adrenaline and noradrenaline are **catecholamines**, and activate **adrenergic** receptors in the effector organs. These receptors are *g-protein-linked* and exist as three types.

1 **α_1-receptors** are linked to G_q and have subtypes α_{1A}, α_{1B} and α_{1D}. Adrenaline and noradrenaline activate α_1-receptors with similar potencies.

2 **α_2-receptors** are linked to $G_{i/o}$ and have subtypes α_{2A}, α_{2B} and α_{2C}. Adrenaline activates α_2-receptors more potently than does noradrenaline.

3 **β-receptors** are linked to G_s and have subtypes β_1, β_2 and β_3. Noradrenaline is more potent than adrenaline at β_1- and β_3-receptors, while adrenaline is more potent at β_2-receptors.

Effects on the heart

Catecholamines acting via cardiac **β_1-receptors** have positive inotropic and chronotropic effects via mechanisms described in Chapters 12 and 13. At rest, cardiac sympathetic nerves exert a tonic accelerating influence on the sinoatrial node, which is, however, overshadowed in younger people by the opposite and dominant effect of parasympathetic vagal tone. Vagal tone decreases progressively with age, causing a rise in the resting heart rate as the sympathetic influence becomes more dominant.

Effects on the vasculature

At rest, vascular sympathetic nerves fire impulses at a rate of 1–2 impulses/s, thereby tonically vasoconstricting the arteries, arterioles and veins. Increasing activation of the sympathetic system causes further vasoconstriction. Vasoconstriction is mediated mainly by α_1-receptors on the vascular smooth muscle cells. The arterial system, particularly the arterioles, is more densely innervated by the sympathetic system than is the venous system. Sympathetic vasoconstriction is particularly marked in the splanchnic, renal, cutaneous and skeletal muscle vascular beds.

The vasculature also contains both β_1- and β_2-receptors, which when stimulated exert a *vasodilating* influence, especially in the *skeletal* and *coronary* circulations. These may have a limited role in dilating these vascular beds in response to adrenaline release, for example during mental stress. In some species, sympathetic *cholinergic* fibres innervate skeletal muscle blood vessels and cause vasodilatation during the defence reaction. A similar but minor role for such nerves in humans has been proposed, but is unproven.

It is a common fallacy that the sympathetic nerves are always activated *en masse*. In reality, changes in sympathetic vasoconstrictor activity can be limited to certain regions (e.g. to the skin during thermoregulation). Similarly, a sympathetically mediated tachycardia occurs with no change in inotropy or vascular resistance during the Bainbridge reflex (see Chapter 27).

The parasympathetic system

The parasympathetic preganglionic neurones involved in regulating the heart have their cell bodies in the **nucleus ambiguus** and the **dorsal motor nucleus** of the medulla. Their axons run in the **vagus** nerve (cranial nerve X) and release acetylcholine onto nicotinic receptors on short postganglionic neurones originating in the cardiac plexus. These innervate the *sinoatrial node (SAN)*, the *atrioventricular node (AVN)* and the *atria*.

Effects on the heart

Basal acetylcholine release by vagal nerve terminals acts on muscarinic receptors to slow the discharge of the SAN. Increased vagal tone further decreases the heart rate and the speed of impulse conduction through the AVN and also decreases the force of atrial contraction when activated.

Effects on the vasculature

Although vagal slowing of the heart can decrease the blood pressure by lowering cardiac output, the parasympathetic system has no effect on total peripheral resistance, because it innervates only a limited number of vascular beds. In particular, activation of parasympathetic fibres in the pelvic nerve causes **erection** by vasodilating arterioles in the erectile tissue of the genitalia. Parasympathetic nerves also cause vasodilatation in the pancreas and salivary glands.

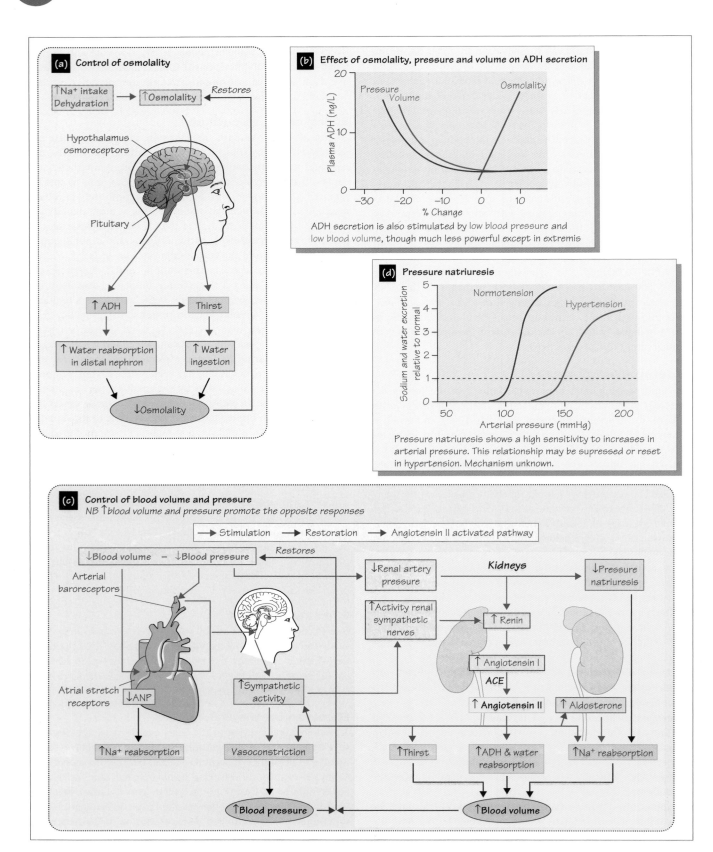

(a) Control of osmolality

↑Na⁺ intake Dehydration → ↑Osmolality ← Restores

Hypothalamus osmoreceptors

Pituitary

↑ADH → Thirst

↑Water reabsorption in distal nephron

↑Water ingestion

↓Osmolality

(b) Effect of osmolality, pressure and volume on ADH secretion

Pressure, Volume, Osmolality

ADH secretion is also stimulated by low blood pressure and low blood volume, though much less powerful except in extremis

(d) Pressure natriuresis

Normotension, Hypertension

Pressure natriuresis shows a high sensitivity to increases in arterial pressure. This relationship may be supressed or reset in hypertension. Mechanism unknown.

(c) Control of blood volume and pressure
NB ↑blood volume and pressure promote the opposite responses

→ Stimulation → Restoration → Angiotensin II activated pathway

↓Blood volume − ↓Blood pressure ← Restores

Arterial baroreceptors

↓Renal artery pressure — Kidneys — ↓Pressure natriuresis

↑Activity renal sympathetic nerves

↑Renin

Atrial stretch receptors ↓ANP

↑Sympathetic activity

↑Angiotensin I

ACE

↑**Angiotensin II** — ↑Aldosterone

↑Na⁺ reabsorption

Vasoconstriction

↑Thirst

↑ADH & water reabsorption

↑Na⁺ reabsorption

↑Blood pressure ← → ↑Blood volume

The Cardiovascular System at a Glance, Fourth Edition. Philip I. Aaronson, Jeremy P.T. Ward, and Michelle J. Connolly.

The baroreceptor system effectively minimizes short-term fluctuations in the arterial blood pressure. Over the longer term, however, the ability to sustain a constant blood pressure depends on maintenance of a *constant blood volume*. This dependency arises because alterations in blood volume affect central venous pressure (CVP) and therefore cardiac output (CO) (see Chapter 17). Changes in CO also ultimately lead to adaptive effects of the vasculature which increase peripheral resistance, and therefore blood pressure (see Chapter 39).

Blood volume is affected by changes in total body Na^+ and water, which are mainly controlled by the kidneys. Maintenance of blood pressure therefore involves mechanisms that adjust renal excretion of Na^+ and water.

Role of sodium and osmoregulation

Alterations in body salt and water content, caused for example by variations in salt or fluid intake or perspiration, result in changes in plasma **osmolality** (see Chapter 5). Any deviation of plasma osmolality from its normal value of *~290 mosmol/kg* is sensed by *hypothalamic osmoreceptors*, which regulate thirst and release of the peptide **antidiuretic hormone** (**ADH**, or *vasopressin*) from the posterior pituitary. ADH enhances reabsorption of water by activating V2 receptors in *principal cells* of the renal collecting duct. This causes **aquaporins** (water channels) to be inserted into their apical membranes, so increasing their permeability to water. Urine is therefore concentrated and water excretion reduced. ADH also affects thirst. Thus, an increase in plasma osmolality due to dehydration causes increased thirst and enhanced release of ADH. Both act to bring plasma osmolality back to normal by restoring body water content (Figure 29a). Opposite effects are stimulated by a reduction in osmolality. ADH secretion is inhibited by alcohol and emotional stress, and strongly stimulated by nausea. Osmoregulation is extremely sensitive to small changes in osmolality (Figure 29b), and normally takes precedence over those controlling blood volume because of the utmost importance of controlling osmolality tightly for cell function (see Chapter 5).

An important consequence of the above is that blood volume is primarily controlled by the Na^+ content of extracellular fluid (ECF), of which plasma is a part. Na^+ and its associated anions Cl^- and HCO_3^- account for about 95% of the osmolality of ECF, thus any change in body Na^+ content (e.g. after eating a salty meal) quickly affects plasma osmolality. The osmoregulatory system responds by readjusting body water content (and therefore plasma volume) in order to restore plasma osmolality. Under normal conditions, therefore, alterations in body Na^+ lead to changes in blood volume. It follows that control of blood volume requires regulation of body (and therefore ECF) Na^+ content, a function carried out by the kidneys.

Control of Na^+ and blood volume by the kidneys

Blood volume directly affects CVP and indirectly affects arterial blood pressure (see Chapter 18). CVP therefore provides a measure of blood volume and is detected by **stretch receptors** primarily in the atria and venoatrial junction. Arterial blood pressure is detected by the **baroreceptors** (see Chapter 27), but directly affects renal function via **pressure natriuresis**. Integration of several mechanisms leads to regulation of Na^+ and therefore blood volume (Figure 29c).

Pressure natriuresis is an intrinsic renal process whereby increases in arterial blood pressure strongly promote diuresis and **natriuresis** (Na^+ excretion in the urine). While the precise mechanisms remain unclear, it is believed that vasodilator prostanoids and nitric oxide increase blood flow in the renal medulla, thereby reducing the osmotic gradient that allows concentration of urine. Na^+ and water reabsorption are therefore suppressed, so more is lost in the urine and blood volume and pressure are restored. Opposite effects occur when pressure is decreased. Pressure natriuresis may be impaired in hypertension (Figure 29d; see Chapter 39).

An increase in blood volume causes stretch of the atria, activating the stretch receptors and also causing release of **atrial natriuretic peptide** (ANP, see below). Increased atrial receptor activity is integrated in the brainstem with baroreceptor activity, and leads to decreased sympathetic outflow to the heart and vasculature and an immediate reduction in arterial blood pressure. Importantly, sympathetic stimulation of the kidney is also reduced, suppressing activity of the **renin – angiotensin – aldosterone** (RAA) **system**; increased renal perfusion pressure does the same. **Renin** is a protease stored in *granular cells* within the juxtaglomerular apparatus. It cleaves the plasma α_2-globulin **angiotensinogen** to form **angiotensin 1**, which is subsequently is converted to the octapeptide **angiotensin 2** by **angiotensin-converting enzyme** (ACE) on the surface of endothelial cells, largely in the lungs. ACE also degrades *bradykinin*, which is why ACE inhibitors cause intractable cough in some patients.

Angiotensin 2 has a number of actions that promote elevation of blood pressure and volume. These include increasing Na^+ reabsorption by the proximal tubule, stimulating thirst, promoting ADH release, increasing activation of the sympathetic nervous system and causing a direct vasoconstriction. Importantly, it also promotes release of the steroid **aldosterone** from the adrenal cortex zona glomerulosa. Aldosterone increases Na^+ reabsorption by principal cells in the distal nephron by stimulating synthesis of basolateral Na^+ pumps and Na^+ channels (**ENaC**) in the apical membrane. It also conserves body Na^+ by enhancing reabsorption from several types of glands, including salivary and sweat glands.

ANP is a 28-amino-acid peptide released from atrial myocytes when they are stretched. ANP causes diuresis and natriuresis by inhibiting ENaC, increasing glomerular filtration rate by dilating renal afferent arterioles, and decreasing renin and aldosterone secretion. It also dilates systemic arterioles and increases capillary permeability. On a cellular level, ANP stimulates membrane-associated guanylyl cyclase and increases intracellular cyclic GMP.

Figure 29c summarizes the response of the above mechanisms to a fall in blood volume and pressure. An elevation would induce the opposite effects.

Although pressure natriuresis has been promoted as the primary mechanism controlling blood volume and long-term blood pressure, more recent evidence suggests that the RAA system may be of predominant importance. This concept is perhaps supported by the effectiveness of ACE inhibitors in clinical practice (e.g. Chapters 38 and 47). ANP and other mechanisms seem to have a more limited role, and may be involved chiefly in the response to volume overload.

Antidiuretic hormone in volume regulation

Under emergency conditions, blood pressure and volume are maintained at the expense of osmoregulation. Thus, a large fall in blood volume or pressure, sensed by the atrial receptors or arterial baroreceptors, causes increased ADH release (Figure 29b) and renal water retention. The ADH system is also rendered more sensitive, so that ADH release is increased at normal osmolality.

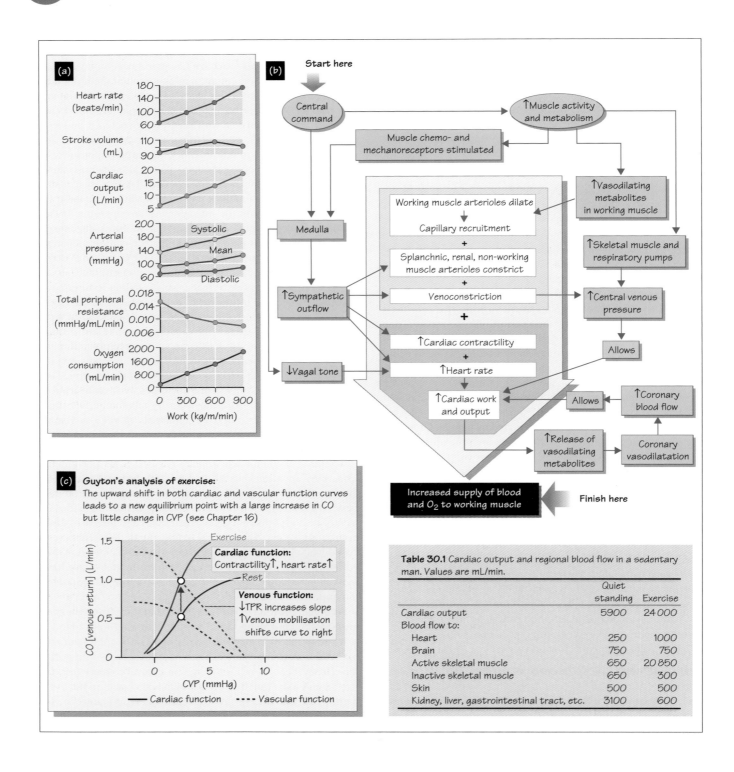

(a)

(b) Start here

(c) Guyton's analysis of exercise:
The upward shift in both cardiac and vascular function curves leads to a new equilibrium point with a large increase in CO but little change in CVP (see Chapter 16)

Cardiac function:
Contractility↑, heart rate↑

Rest

Venous function:
↓TPR increases slope
↑Venous mobilisation shifts curve to right

— Cardiac function   ---- Vascular function

Table 30.1 Cardiac output and regional blood flow in a sedentary man. Values are mL/min.

	Quiet standing	Exercise
Cardiac output	5900	24 000
Blood flow to:		
Heart	250	1000
Brain	750	750
Active skeletal muscle	650	20 850
Inactive skeletal muscle	650	300
Skin	500	500
Kidney, liver, gastrointestinal tract, etc.	3100	600

Figure 30a summarizes important cardiovascular adaptations that occur at increasing levels of dynamic (rhythmic) exercise, thereby allowing working muscles to be supplied with the increased amount of O_2 they require. By far the most important of these adaptations is an increase in cardiac output (CO), which rises almost linearly with the rate of muscle O_2 consumption (level of work) as a result of increases in both *heart rate* and to a lesser extent *stroke volume*. The heart rate is accelerated by a reduction in vagal tone, and by

The Cardiovascular System at a Glance, Fourth Edition. Philip I. Aaronson, Jeremy P.T. Ward, and Michelle J. Connolly.

increases in sympathetic nerve firing and circulating catecholamines. The resulting stimulation of cardiac β-adrenoceptors increases stroke volume by *increasing myocardial contractility* and enabling more complete systolic emptying of the ventricles. CO is the limiting factor determining the maximum exercise capacity.

Table 30.1 shows that the increased CO is channelled mainly to the active muscles, which may receive 85% of CO against about 15–20% at rest, and to the heart. This is caused by a profound arteriolar vasodilatation in these organs. Dilatation of terminal arterioles causes **capillary recruitment**, a large increase in the number of open capillaries, which shortens the diffusion distance between capillaries and muscle fibres. This, combined with increases in P_{CO_2}, temperature and acidity, promotes the release of O_2 from haemoglobin, allowing skeletal muscle to increase its O_2 extraction from the basal level of 25–30% to about 90% during maximal exercise.

Increased firing of sympathetic nerves and levels of circulating catecholamines constrict arterioles in the *splanchnic* and *renal* vascular beds, and in *non-exercising muscle*, reducing the blood flow to these organs. Cutaneous blood flow is also initially reduced. As core body temperature rises, however, cutaneous blood flow increases as autonomically mediated vasodilatation occurs to promote cooling (see Chapter 25). With very strenuous exercise, cutaneous perfusion again falls as vasoconstriction diverts blood to the muscles. Blood flow to the crucial cerebral vasculature remains constant.

Vasodilatation of the skeletal and cutaneous vascular beds decreases total peripheral resistance (TPR). This is sufficient to balance the effect of the increased CO on diastolic blood pressure, which rises only slightly and may even fall, depending on the balance between skeletal muscle vasodilatation and splanchnic/renal vasoconstriction. However, significant rises in the systolic and pulse pressures are caused by the more rapid and forceful ejection of blood by the left ventricle, leading to some elevation of the mean arterial blood pressure.

Any increase in CO must of course be accompanied by an increase in venous return, which is supported by venoconstriction and the action of skeletal muscle and respiratory pumps. Coupled with the fall in TPR, these actions allow a large increase in CO with little change in CVP (Figure 30c; see Chapter 17).

Effects of exercise on plasma volume

Arteriolar dilatation in skeletal muscles increases capillary hydrostatic pressure, while capillary recruitment vastly increases the surface area of the microcirculation available to exchange fluid. These effects, coupled with a rise in interstitial osmolarity caused by an increased production of metabolites within the muscle fibres, lead via the Starling mechanism to *extravasation of fluid into muscles* (Chapter 20). Taking into account also fluid losses caused by sweating, plasma volume may decrease by 15% during strenuous exercise. This fluid loss is partially compensated by enhanced fluid reabsorption in the vasoconstricted vascular beds, where capillary pressure decreases.

Regulation and coordination of the cardiovascular adaptation to exercise

In anticipation of exercise, and during its initial stages, a process termed **central command** (Figure 30b, upper left) initiates the cardiovascular adaptations necessary for increased effort. Impulses from the cerebral cortex act on the medulla to suppress vagal tone, thereby increasing the heart rate and CO. Central command is also thought to raise the set point of the baroreceptor reflex. This allows the blood pressure to be regulated around a higher set point, resulting in an increased sympathetic outflow which contributes to the rise in CO and causes constriction of the splanchnic and renal circulations. An increase in circulating adrenaline also vasodilates skeletal muscle arterioles via β2-receptors. The magnitude of these anticipatory effects increases in proportion to the degree of perceived effort.

As exercise continues, cardiovascular regulation by central command is supplemented by two further control systems which are activated and become crucial. These involve: (i) autonomic reflexes (Figure 30b, left); and (ii) direct effects of metabolites generated locally in working skeletal and cardiac muscle (right).

Systemic effects mediated by autonomic reflexes

Nervous impulses originating mainly from receptors in working muscle which respond to contraction (mechanoreceptors) and locally generated metabolites and ischaemia (chemoreceptors) are carried to the CNS via afferent nerves. CNS autonomic control centres respond by suppressing vagal tone and causing graded increases in sympathetic outflow which are matched to the ongoing level of exercise. An increased release of adrenaline and noradrenaline from the adrenal glands causes plasma catecholamines to rise by as much as 10- to 20-fold.

Effects of local metabolites on muscle and heart

The autonomic reflexes described above are responsible for most of the cardiac and vasoconstricting adaptations to exercise. However, the marked vasodilatation of coronary and skeletal muscle arterioles is almost entirely caused by *local metabolites* generated in the heart and working skeletal muscle. This **metabolic hyperaemia** (see Chapter 23) causes decreased vascular resistance and increased blood flow. Capillary recruitment (see above) is an important consequence of metabolic hyperaemia.

Static exercises such as lifting and carrying involve maintained muscle contractions with no joint movement. This results in vascular compression and a decreased muscle blood flow, leading to a build-up of muscle metabolites. These activate muscle chemoreceptors, resulting in a *pressor reflex* involving *tachycardia*, and *increases* in *CO* and *TPR*. The resulting rise in blood pressure is much greater than in dynamic exercise causing the same rise in O_2 consumption.

Effects of training

Athletic training has effects on the cardiovascular system that improve delivery of O_2 to muscle cells, allowing them to work harder. The ventricular walls thicken and the cavities become larger, increasing the stroke volume from about 75 to 120 mL. The resting heart rate may fall as low as 45 beats/min, due to an increase in vagal tone, while the maximal rate remains near 180 beats/min. These changes allow CO, the crucial determinant of exercise capacity, to increase more during strenuous exercise, reaching levels of 35 L/min or more. TPR falls, in part due to a decreased sympathetic outflow. The capillary density of skeletal muscle increases, and the muscle fibres contain more mitochondria, promoting oxygen extraction and utilization.

31 Shock and haemorrhage

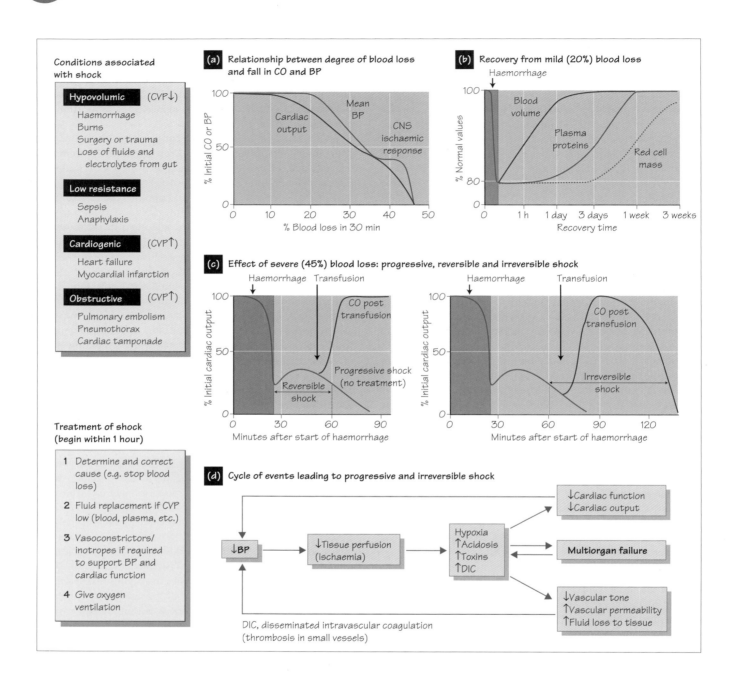

Conditions associated with shock

Hypovolumic (CVP↓)
- Haemorrhage
- Burns
- Surgery or trauma
- Loss of fluids and electrolytes from gut

Low resistance
- Sepsis
- Anaphylaxis

Cardiogenic (CVP↑)
- Heart failure
- Myocardial infarction

Obstructive (CVP↑)
- Pulmonary embolism
- Pneumothorax
- Cardiac tamponade

Treatment of shock (begin within 1 hour)

1. Determine and correct cause (e.g. stop blood loss)
2. Fluid replacement if CVP low (blood, plasma, etc.)
3. Vasoconstrictors/inotropes if required to support BP and cardiac function
4. Give oxygen ventilation

(a) Relationship between degree of blood loss and fall in CO and BP

(b) Recovery from mild (20%) blood loss

(c) Effect of severe (45%) blood loss: progressive, reversible and irreversible shock

(d) Cycle of events leading to progressive and irreversible shock

DIC, disseminated intravascular coagulation (thrombosis in small vessels)

Cardiovascular or **circulatory shock** refers to an acute condition where there is a generalized inadequacy of blood flow throughout the body. The patient appears pale, grey or cyanotic, with cold clammy skin, a weak rapid pulse and rapid shallow breathing. Urine output is reduced and blood pressure (BP) is generally low. Conscious patients may develop intense thirst. Cardiovascular shock may be caused by a reduced blood volume (**hypovolaemic shock**), profound vasodilatation (**low-resistance shock**), acute failure of the heart to maintain output (**cardiogenic shock**) or blockage of the cardiopulmonary circuit (e.g. pulmonary embolism).

Haemorrhagic shock

Blood loss (**haemorrhage**) is the most common cause of **hypovolaemic** shock. Loss of up to ~20% of total blood volume is unlikely to elicit shock in a fit person. If 20–30% of blood volume is lost, shock is normally induced and blood pressure may be depressed, although death is not common. Loss of 30–50% of volume, however, causes

The Cardiovascular System at a Glance, Fourth Edition. Philip I. Aaronson, Jeremy P.T. Ward, and Michelle J. Connolly.

a profound reduction in BP and cardiac output (Figure 31a), with severe shock which may become **irreversible** or **refractory** (see below). Severity is related to amount and rate of blood loss – a very rapid loss of 30% can be fatal, whereas 50% over 24 h may be survived. Above 50% death is generally inevitable.

Immediate compensation

The initial fall in BP is detected by the **baroreceptors**, and reduced blood flow activates peripheral **chemoreceptors**. These cause a reflex increase in sympathetic and decrease in parasympathetic drive, with a subsequent increase in heart rate, venoconstriction (which restores central venous pressure, CVP) and vasoconstriction of the splanchnic, cutaneous, renal and skeletal muscle circulations which helps restore BP. Vasoconstriction leads to pallor, reduced urine production and lactic acidosis. Increased sympathetic discharge also results in sweating, and characteristic clammy skin. Sympathetic vasoconstriction of the renal artery plus reduced renal artery pressure stimulates the **renin–angiotensin system** (see Chapter 29), and production of **angiotensin II**, a powerful vasoconstrictor. This has an important role in the recovery of BP and stimulates thirst. In more severe blood loss, reduction in atrial stretch receptor output stimulates production of **vasopressin** (antidiuretic hormone, **ADH**) and adrenal production of **adrenaline**, both of which contribute to vasoconstriction. These initial mechanisms may prevent any significant fall in BP or cardiac output following moderate blood loss, even though the degree of shock may be serious. If BP falls below 50 mmHg the **CNS ischaemic response** is activated, with powerful sympathetic activation (Figure 31a).

Medium- and long-term mechanisms

The vasoconstriction and/or fall in BP decreases capillary hydrostatic pressure, resulting in fluid movement from the interstitium back into the vasculature (see Chapter 21). This 'internal transfusion' may increase blood volume by ~0.5 L and takes hours to develop. Increased glucose production by the liver may contribute by raising plasma and interstitial fluid osmolarity, thus drawing water from intracellular compartments. This process results in haemodilution, and patients with severe shock often present with a reduced haematocrit. Fluid volume is brought back to normal over days by increased fluid intake (thirst), decreased urine production (**oliguria**) due to renal vasoconstriction, increased Na^+ reabsorption caused by the production of **aldosterone** (stimulated by angiotensin II) and a fall in atrial natriuretic peptide (**ANP**), and increased water reabsorption caused by vasopressin (Figure 31b). The liver replaces plasma proteins within a week, and haematocrit returns to normal within 6 weeks due to stimulation of **erythropoiesis** (Figure 31b; see Chapter 6).

Other responses to haemorrhage are *increased ventilation* due to reduced flow through **chemoreceptors** (carotid body) and/or acidosis; *decreased blood coagulation time* due to an increase in platelets and fibrinogen that occurs within minutes (see Chapter 7); and *increased white cell (neutrophil) count* after 2–5 h.

Complications and irreversible (refractory) shock

When blood loss exceeds 30%, cardiac output may temporarily improve before continuing to decline (**progressive shock**; Figure 31c). This is due to a vicious circle initiated by circulatory failure and tissue hypoxia/ischaemia, leading to acidosis, toxin release and eventually **multiorgan failure**, including **depression of cardiac muscle function**, acute respiratory distress syndrome (**ARDS**), **renal failure**, disseminated intravascular coagulation (**DIC**), **hepatic failure** and damage to **intestinal mucosa**. Increased vascular permeability further decreases blood volume due to fluid loss into the tissues, and vascular tone is depressed. These complications lead to further tissue damage, impairment of tissue perfusion and gas exchange (Figure 31d). Rapid treatment (e.g. transfusion) is essential; after 1 h ('*the golden hour*') mortality increases sharply if the patient is still in shock, as transfusion and vasoconstrictor drugs may then cause only a temporary respite before cardiac output falls irrevocably. This is called **irreversible** or **refractory** shock (Figure 31c), and is primarily related to irretrievable damage to the heart.

Other types of hypovolaemic shock

Severe burns result in a loss of plasma in exudate from damaged tissue. As red cells are not lost, there is **haemoconcentration**, which will increase blood viscosity. Treatment of burns-related shock therefore involves infusion of plasma rather than whole blood. **Traumatic and surgical shock** can occur after major injury or surgery. Although this is partly due to external blood loss, blood and plasma can also be lost into the tissues, and there may be dehydration. **Other conditions** include severe diarrhoea or vomiting and loss of Na^+ (e.g. **cholera**) with a consequent reduction in blood volume even if water is given, unless electrolytes are replenished.

Low-resistance shock

Unlike in hypovolaemic shock, patients with low-resistance shock may present with warm skin due to profound peripheral vasodilatation.

Septic shock is caused by a profound vasodilatation due to endotoxins released by infecting bacteria, partly via induction of inducible nitric oxide synthase (see Chapter 24). Capillary permeability and cardiac function may be impaired, with consequent loss of fluid to the tissues and depressed cardiac output.

Anaphylactic shock is a rapidly developing and life-threatening condition resulting from presentation of antigen to a sensitized individual (e.g. bee stings or peanut allergy). A severe **allergic reaction** may result, with release of large amounts of histamine. This causes profound vasodilatation, and increased microvasculature permeability, leading to protein and fluid loss to tissues (oedema). Rapid treatment with antihistamines and glucocorticoids is necessary, but immediate application of a vasoconstrictor (adrenaline) may be required to save the patient's life.

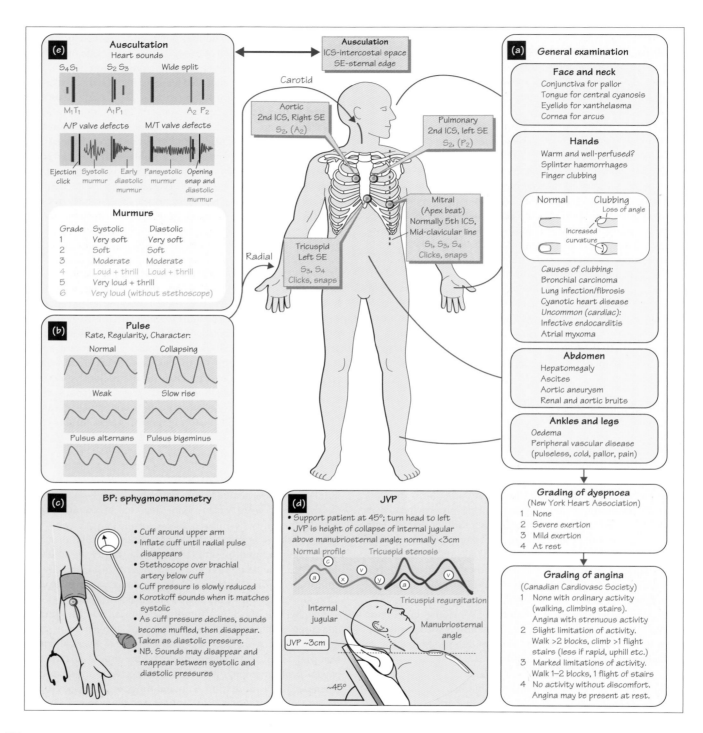

(e) Auscultation
Heart sounds

$S_4 S_1$ $S_2 S_3$ Wide split

$M_1 T_1$ $A_1 P_1$ $A_2 P_2$

A/P valve defects   M/T valve defects

Ejection click   Systolic murmur   Early diastolic murmur   Pansystolic murmur   Opening snap and diastolic murmur

Murmurs

Grade	Systolic	Diastolic
1	Very soft	Very soft
2	Soft	Soft
3	Moderate	Moderate
4	Loud + thrill	Loud + thrill
5	Very loud + thrill	
6	Very loud (without stethoscope)	

Ausculation
ICS-intercostal space
SE-sternal edge

Carotid

Aortic
2nd ICS, Right SE
S_2, (A_2)

Pulmonary
2nd ICS, left SE
S_2, (P_2)

Mitral
(Apex beat)
Normally 5th ICS,
Mid-clavicular line
S_1, S_3, S_4
Clicks, snaps

Radial

Tricuspid
Left SE
S_3, S_4
Clicks, snaps

(a) General examination

Face and neck
Conjunctiva for pallor
Tongue for central cyanosis
Eyelids for xanthelasma
Cornea for arcus

Hands
Warm and well-perfused?
Splinter haemorrhages
Finger clubbing

Normal   Clubbing
Loss of angle
Increased curvature

Causes of clubbing:
Bronchial carcinoma
Lung infection/fibrosis
Cyanotic heart disease
Uncommon (cardiac):
Infective endocarditis
Atrial myxoma

Abdomen
Hepatomegaly
Ascites
Aortic aneurysm
Renal and aortic bruits

Ankles and legs
Oedema
Peripheral vascular disease
(pulseless, cold, pallor, pain)

(b) Pulse
Rate, Regularity, Character:

Normal   Collapsing

Weak   Slow rise

Pulsus alternans   Pulsus bigeminus

(c) BP: sphygmomanometry

- Cuff around upper arm
- Inflate cuff until radial pulse disappears
- Stethoscope over brachial artery below cuff
- Cuff pressure is slowly reduced
- Korotkoff sounds when it matches systolic
- As cuff pressure declines, sounds become muffled, then disappear. Taken as diastolic pressure.
- NB. Sounds may disappear and reappear between systolic and diastolic pressures

(d) JVP

- Support patient at 45°; turn head to left
- JVP is height of collapse of internal jugular above manubriosternal angle; normally <3cm

Normal profile   Tricuspid stenosis

Tricuspid regurgitation

Internal jugular   Manubriosternal angle

JVP ~3cm

~45°

Grading of dyspnoea
(New York Heart Association)
1 None
2 Severe exertion
3 Mild exertion
4 At rest

Grading of angina
(Canadian Cardiovasc Society)
1 None with ordinary activity (walking, climbing stairs). Angina with strenuous activity
2 Slight limitation of activity. Walk >2 blocks, climb >1 flight stairs (less if rapid, uphill etc.)
3 Marked limitations of activity. Walk 1–2 blocks, 1 flight of stairs
4 No activity without discomfort. Angina may be present at rest.

History

Presenting complaint The reason the patient has sought medical attention. Most common in cardiovascular disease are chest pain, dyspnoea (breathlessness), palpitations and syncope (dizziness).

History of presenting complaint Explore features of the presenting complaint (e.g. onset, progression, severity; Figure 32a).

- **Dyspnoea:** the commonest symptom of heart disease. Establish whether it occurs at rest, on exertion, on lying flat (**orthopnoea**) or at night. Determine rate of onset (sudden, gradual). Dyspnoea due to pulmonary oedema (heart failure) may cause sudden wakening (**paroxysmal nocturnal dyspnoea, PND**), a frightening experience in which the patient wakes at night, gasping for breath.

The Cardiovascular System at a Glance, Fourth Edition. Philip I. Aaronson, Jeremy P.T. Ward, and Michelle J. Connolly.

- **Chest pain 'SOCRATES'**
Site: where is it? **O**nset: gradual, sudden? **C**haracter: sharp, dull, crushing? **R**adiation: to arm, neck, jaw? **A**ssociated symptoms: dyspnoea, sweating, nausea, syncope or palpitations? **T**iming: duration of the pain? Is it constant or does it come and go? **E**xacerbating and relieving factors: worse/better with breathing, posture? **S**everity: does it interfere with daily activities or sleep? **Angina** is described as crushing central chest pain, radiating to left arm/shoulder, back, neck or jaw. Pain due to **pericarditis** is sharp and severe, aggravated by inspiration, and is classically relieved by leaning forward.
- **Palpitations:** increased awareness of the heart beat. Ask patient to tap out the rhythm. Premature beats and extrasystoles give sensation of **missed beats**.
- **Syncope:** commonly **vasovagal**, provoked by anxiety or standing for extended periods of time. Cardiovascular syncope is usually due to sudden changes in heart rhythm; for example, heart block, paroxysmal arrhythmias (**Stokes–Adams attacks**).
- **Others:** fatigue – heart failure, arrhythmias and drugs (e.g. β-blockers). Oedema and abdominal discomfort – raised central venous pressure (CVP), heart failure. Leg pain on walking may be due to **claudication** secondary to peripheral vascular disease.

Past medical history Previous and current conditions. Ask about myocardial infarction (MI), stroke, hypertension, diabetes, rheumatic fever. Also recent blood pressure measurements and lipid levels, and any investigations.

Drug history Prescribed and over-the-counter medications. Ascertain compliance. Ask about **drug allergies** and their effect(s).

Family, occupational and social history Family history of MI, hypertension, diabetes, stroke or sudden death? **Smoking** including duration and amount and alcohol consumption. **Occupation:** stress, sedentary or active.

Examination

General examination (Figure 32a)
Assess general appearance: obesity, cachexia (wasting), jaundice. Note the presence of scars; for example, a sternotomy scar in the midline (coronary artery bypass graft, CABG; valve replacement). NB: if a midline sternotomy scar is present, inspect the legs for a saphenous vein graft scar.
- **Hands:** warm and well-perfused or cold? Peripheral cyanosis (dusky blue discoloration, deoxyhaemoglobin >5 g/dL, e.g. vasoconstriction, shock, heart failure; not seen in anaemia); assess capillary refill by pressing on the nail bed for 5 s and releasing. Normal capillary refill is <2 s. Inspect nails for clubbing (Figure 32a), tar stains, splinter haemorrhages (infective endocarditis). Inspect the finger pads for Janeway lesions and Osler's nodes (infective endocarditis).
- **Pulses:** radial pulse; assess rate and character (regular or irregular). Feel for a collapsing pulse (aortic regurgitation).
- **Blood pressure:** measure the blood pressure over the brachial artery (ideally in both arms and take the highest reading).
- **Face and neck:** determine whether or not the jugular venous pressure (JVP) is raised. It is raised if the tip of the pulsation in the internal jugular vein is >3 cm above the angle of Louis. Feel the carotid pulse and assess its volume and character. Inspect the conjunctivae for pallor (anaemia); cornea for corneal arcus (hyperlipidaemia, although normal in old age); eyelids for xanthelasma (soft yellow plaques: hyperlipidaemia); tongue for central cyanosis; dental hygiene (infective endocarditis); cheeks for malar flush (mitral valve disease); retinae for hypertensive or diabetic retinopathy.

Examination of the praecordium
- **Palpation: apex beat**, usually at fifth intercostal space, midclavicular line (mitral area). *Non-palpable*: obesity, hyperinflation, pleural effusion. *Displaced*: cardiomegaly, dilated cardiomyopathy, pneumothorax. *Tapping*: mitral stenosis. *Double*: ventricular hypertrophy. *Heaving* (forceful and sustained): pressure overload – hypertension, aortic stenosis. *Parasternal heave*: right ventricular hypertrophy. **Thrills** are palpable (therefore strong) murmurs (see below).
- **Auscultation** (Figure 32e; see Chapters 14, 52–54): correlate with radial or carotid pulse. **First heart sound (S₁):** closure of mitral and tricuspid valves. *Loud*: atrioventricular valve stenosis, short PR interval; *soft*: mitral regurgitation, long PR interval, heart failure. **Second heart sound (S₂):** closure of aortic (A₂) and pulmonary (P₂) valves, A₂ louder and preceding P₂. *Loud A₂/P₂*: systemic/pulmonary hypertension. *Splitting*: normal during inspiration or exercise, particularly in the young. *Wide splitting*: delayed activation (e.g. right bundle branch block) or termination (pulmonary hypertension, stenosis) of RV systole. *Reverse splitting*: delayed activation (e.g. left bundle branch block) or termination (hypertension, aortic stenosis) of LV systole. **Others: S₃** – rapid ventricular filling, common in the young but may reflect heart failure in patients >30 years. **S₄** – precedes S₁, due to ventricular stiffness and abnormal filling during atrial systole. Presence of S₃ and/or S₄ gives a **gallop rhythm**. **Ejection click**: after S₁, opening of stenotic semilunar valve. **Opening snap**: after S₂, opening of stenotic atrioventricular valve.
- **Murmurs** (Figure 32e): added sounds due to turbulent blood flow. Soft systolic murmurs are common and innocent in young (~40% children 3–8 years) and in exercise; **diastolic murmurs** are pathological. Most non-benign murmurs are due to **valve defects** (see Chapters 53 and 54). Others include a hyperdynamic circulation and atrial or ventricular septal defects.
- **Abdomen:** palpate for liver enlargement (**hepatomegaly**), ascites (raised CVP, heart failure), splenomegaly (infective endocarditis). The **abdominal aorta** is pulsatile in thin individuals but not expansile (indicates **abdominal aortic aneurysm**).
- **Lower limbs:** pitting oedema, peripheral vascular disease.

Pulse (Figure 32b)
Resting rate 60–90 beats/min, slows with age and fitness. Compare radial with apex beat (delay: e.g. atrial fibrillation) and femoral/lower limbs (delay: atherosclerosis, aortic stenosis). Changes in rate with breathing are normal (**sinus arrhythmia**).
- **Irregular beats** *Regularly irregular*: e.g. extrasystoles (disappear on exertion), second-degree heart block. *Irregularly irregular*: e.g. atrial fibrillation (unchanged by exertion).
- **Character** (carotid): *thready or weak*: heart failure, shock, valve disease; *slow rising*: aortic stenosis. *Bounding*: high output; followed by *sharp fall* (**collapsing**): very high output, aortic valve regurgitation. *Alternating weak–strong* (**pulsus alternans**): left heart failure; distinguish from **pulsus bigeminus**, normal beat followed by weak premature beat. *Pulsus paradoxus, accentuated weakening of pulse on inspiration*: cardiac tamponade, severe asthma, restrictive pericarditis.

Blood pressure (Figure 32c)
At rest, adult arterial systolic pressure is normally <140 mmHg, diastolic <90 mmHg. Systolic rises with age.
- **JVP** (Figure 32d): Indirect measure of right atrial pressure. Raised in heart failure and volume overload. Large 'a' wave (see Chapter 16): pulmonary hypertension, pulmonary valve stenosis, tricuspid stenosis; large 'v' wave: tricuspid regurgitation. Absent 'a' wave: atrial fibrillation.

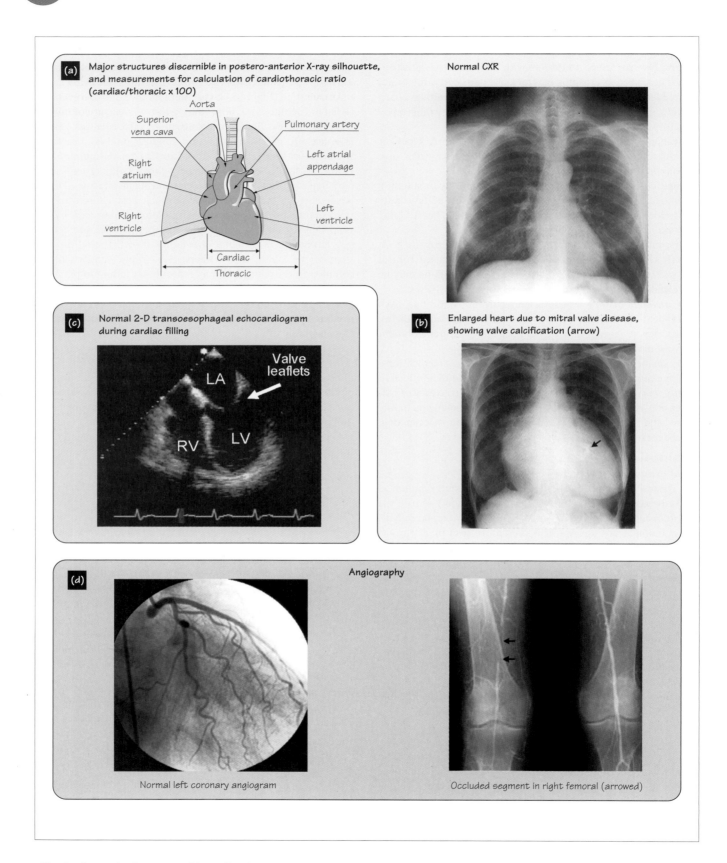

(a) Major structures discernible in postero-anterior X-ray silhouette, and measurements for calculation of cardiothoracic ratio (cardiac/thoracic x 100)

- Aorta
- Superior vena cava
- Right atrium
- Pulmonary artery
- Left atrial appendage
- Right ventricle
- Left ventricle
- Cardiac
- Thoracic

Normal CXR

(c) Normal 2-D transoesophageal echocardiogram during cardiac filling

Valve leaflets

LA
RV LV

(b) Enlarged heart due to mitral valve disease, showing valve calcification (arrow)

Angiography

(d)

Normal left coronary angiogram

Occluded segment in right femoral (arrowed)

The Cardiovascular System at a Glance, Fourth Edition. Philip I. Aaronson, Jeremy P.T. Ward, and Michelle J. Connolly.

Key investigations for cardiovascular disease are the electrocardiogram (ECG; see Chapter 14), chest X-ray and echocardiogram. Others include exercise ECG testing, ambulatory blood pressure monitoring, lipid profile, cardiac enzyme assays and catheterization with coronary or pulmonary angiography.

X-rays (chest radiography)

The chest X-ray (CXR) is an essential diagnostic tool. The initial CXR is taken in the postero-anterior (PA) direction, with the patient upright and at full inspiration. Figure 33a shows the major structures in which gross abnormalities can be detected, such as enlargement of the heart chambers and major vessels, and a normal PA CXR. Heart size and **cardiothoracic ratio** (size of heart relative to thoracic cavity) can also be estimated. This ratio is normally <50%, except in neonates, infants and athletes, but may be greatly increased in heart failure (see Chapter 46). Calcification due to tissue damage and necrosis may be detected by CXR if significant (Figure 33c). Enlargement of the main pulmonary arteries coupled with pruning of the peripheral arteries suggests pulmonary hypertension, whereas haziness of the lung fields is indicative of pulmonary venous hypertension and fluid accumulation in the tissues.

Echocardiography and Doppler ultrasound

Echocardiography can be used to detect enlarged hearts and abnormal cardiac movement, and to estimate the ejection fraction. An ultrasound pulse of ~2.5 MHz is generated by a piezoelectric transmitter–receiver on the chest wall, and is reflected back by internal structures. As sound travels through fluid at a known velocity, the time taken between transmission and reception is a measure of distance. This allows a picture of internal structure to be built up. In an M-mode echocardiogram the transmitter remains static, and the trace shows changes in reflections with time. In two-dimensional (2D) echocardiograms the transmitter scans backwards and forwards, so that a 2D picture is built up. Echocardiography is non-invasive and quick. However, when imaging the heart it is restricted by the presence of the rib cage and air in the lungs, which reflect or absorb the ultrasound. This interference can be minimized by using specific locations on the chest. Alternatively, the probe can be placed in the oesophagus (**transoesophageal echocardiography**, TOE). Although more invasive, this provides greater resolution (Figure 33b) and improved access to pulmonary artery, aorta and atria.

Sound reflected back from a moving target shows a shift in frequency; for example, if the target is moving towards the source, the frequency is increased. This **Doppler** effect can be used to calculate the *velocity* of blood movement from the frequency shift in the ultrasound pulse caused by reflection from red cells, and the *pressure gradient* across obstructions from the Bernoulli equation: $P = 4 \times (\text{velocity})^2$. Blood flow can be calculated if the cross-sectional area of the vessel is estimated using echocardiography.

Catheterization and angiography

Radiopaque catheters (opaque to X-rays) are introduced into the heart or blood vessels via peripheral veins or arteries. Catheters with small balloons at the tip (**Swan–Ganz** catheters) assist placement from the venous side as the tip moves with the flow. Placement can be ascertained from the pressure wave-form and X-rays. Catheters are used for measurement of pressures or cardiac output, for **angiography**, or to take samples for estimating metabolites and P_{O_2}. Left atrial pressure cannot be measured directly as it requires access via the mitral valve. Instead, a Swan–Ganz catheter is passed through the right heart, and is wedged in a distal pulmonary artery. As there is thus no flow through that artery, the pressure is the same throughout the capillaries to the pulmonary vein. This **pulmonary wedge pressure** is an estimate of left atrial pressure.

Angiography A radiopaque **contrast medium** is introduced into the lumen of cardiac chambers, and coronary (Figure 33d), pulmonary or other blood vessels. This allows direct visualization of the blood and vessels with X-rays, and can be used to examine cardiac pumping function and to locate blockages (e.g. emboli) in the vasculature (Figure 33d).

Imaging

Advances in medical imaging techniques have provided several powerful diagnostic aids of particular use in cardiac disease.

Nuclear imaging Radiopharmaceuticals introduced into the heart or circulation are detected by a gamma camera, and their distribution (depending on type) can be used to measure or detect cardiac muscle perfusion, damage and function. Three-dimensional information can be obtained in a similar fashion using single photon emission computed tomography (**SPECT**). The most common tracers used are thallium-201 (^{201}Tl), and technetium-99m (^{99m}Tc) labelled sestamibi (a large synthetic molecule of the isonitrile family), which are distributed according to blood flow and taken up by living cardiac muscle cells. These therefore show up brightly immediately after infusion; ischaemic and infarcted areas remain dark because of poor perfusion. Whereas over time ^{201}Tl will redistribute into ischaemic areas as well, ^{99m}Tcsestamibi will not, so a delayed ^{201}Tl image will show infarcted areas only. This is useful for determining savable areas of the heart prior to angioplasty or coronary bypass. However, ^{99m}Tc has a higher photon energy and shorter half-life, allowing lower radionucleotide doses with better images. It is therefore better for SPECT, and the higher energy allows **gated acquisition** (sequential images taken during a cardiac cycle), and evaluation of resting left and right ventricular function in combination with either resting or exercise myocardial perfusion.

Magnetic resonance imaging (MRI) Radiofrequency stimulation of hydrogen atoms held in a high magnetic field emits energy, which can be used to generate a high-fidelity image that reflects tissue density, MRI is useful for the location of masses and malformations, including aneurysms. It is entirely non-invasive and uses no damaging radiations.

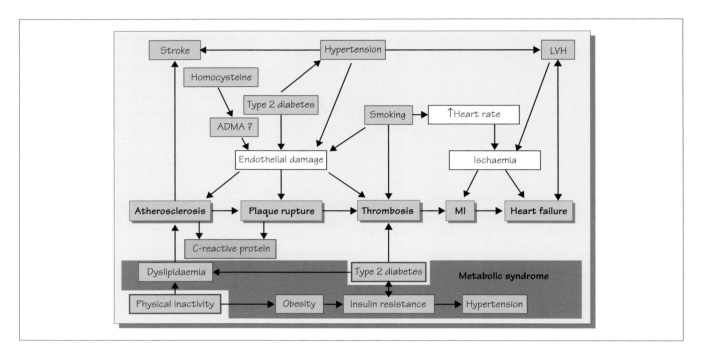

The main manifestations of cardiovascular disease (CVD) are coronary heart disease (CHD), cerebrovascular disease (stroke) and peripheral vascular disease, and the underlying cause of these is most often atherosclerosis (see Chapter 37). Numerous factors or conditions are known to increase (or decrease) the probability that atherosclerosis will develop, and the presence in an individual of these **cardiovascular risk factors** can be used to assess the likelihood that overt cardiovascular morbidity and death will occur in the medium term. Table 34.1 presents an abbreviated summary of the impact of major risk factors on CHD as determined by the Framingham Heart Study.

Some risk factors such as *age*, *male sex* and *family history of CVD* are **fixed**. However, others, including *dyslipidaemias, smoking, hypertension, diabetes mellitus, obesity* and *physical inactivity*, are **modifiable.** These probably account for over 90% of the risk of developing atherosclerotic CVD. The attempt to prevent CVD by targeting modifiable risk factors has become a cornerstone of modern disease management because the occurrence of overt CVD is preceded by the development of subclinical atherosclerosis which takes many years to progress.

Figure 34 illustrates the main mechanisms by which major risk factors are thought to promote the development of atherosclerosis and its most important consequence, CHD. Additional aspects of dyslipidaemias and hypertension are described in Chapters 36–39.

Modifiable risk factors

Dyslipidaemias are a heterogeneous group of conditions characterized by abnormal levels of one or more **lipoproteins**. Lipoproteins are blood-borne particles that contain cholesterol and other lipids. They function to transfer lipids between the intestines, liver and other organs (see Chapter 36).

Table 34.1 Major modifiable risk factors: effects on the risk of coronary heart disease in men and women aged 35–64 years.

Risk factors	Age-adjusted relative risk*	
	Men	Women
Cholesterol >240 mg/dL	1.9	1.8
Hypertension >140/90 mmHg	2.0	2.2
Diabetes	1.5	3.7
Left ventricular hypertrophy	3.0	4.6
Smoking	1.5	1.1

* Indicates relative risk for individuals with a given factor compared with those without it.

Dyslipidaemias involving excessive plasma concentrations of **low-density lipoprotein (LDL)** are associated with rises in plasma cholesterol levels, because LDL contains 70% of total plasma cholesterol. As the level of plasma cholesterol rises, particularly above 240 mg/dL (6.2 mmol/L), there is a progressive increase in the risk of CVD due to the attendant rise in LDL levels. LDL has a pivotal role in causing atherosclerosis because it can be converted to an oxidized form, which damages the vascular wall (see Chapter 37). Drugs that lower plasma LDL (and therefore oxidized LDL) slow the progression of atherosclerosis and reduce the occurrence of CVD. Elevated levels of **lipoprotein (a)**, a form of LDL containing the unique protein **apo(a)**, have been reported to confer additional cardiovascular risk. Apo(a) contains a structural component closely resembling plasminogen, and it may inhibit fibrinolysis (see Chapters 8 and 45) by competing with plasminogen for endogenous activators.

On the other hand, the risk of CVD is *inversely* related to the plasma concentration of **high-density lipoprotein (HDL)**, possibly because HDL functions to remove cholesterol from body tissues,

The Cardiovascular System at a Glance, Fourth Edition. Philip I. Aaronson, Jeremy P.T. Ward, and Michelle J. Connolly.

and may act to inhibit lipoprotein oxidation. The ratio of total to HDL cholesterol is therefore a better predictor of risk than cholesterol levels per se. Low HDL levels often coexist with high levels of plasma **triglycerides**, which are also correlated with CVD. This is probably due to the atherogenicity of the triglyceride-rich **very low-density lipoprotein (VLDL)** and **intermediate-density lipoprotein (IDL)**.

Hypertension, defined as a blood pressure above 140/90 mmHg, occurs in ~25% of the population, and in more than half of people who are middle aged or older. Hypertension promotes atherogenesis, probably by damaging the endothelium and causing other deleterious effects on the walls of large arteries. Hypertension damages blood vessels of the brain and kidneys, increasing the risk of stroke and renal failure. The higher cardiac workload imposed by the increased arterial pressure also causes a thickening of the left ventricular wall. This process, termed **left ventricular hypertrophy (LVH)**, is both a cause and harbinger of more serious cardiovascular damage. LVH predisposes the myocardium to arrhythmias and ischaemia, and is a major contributor to heart failure, myocardial infarction (MI) and sudden death.

Physical inactivity promotes CVD via multiple mechanisms. Low fitness is associated with reduced plasma HDL, higher levels of blood pressure and insulin resistance, and **obesity**, itself a CVD risk factor. Studies show that a moderate to high level of fitness is associated with a halving of CVD mortality.

Diabetes mellitus is a metabolic disease present in approximately 5% of the population. Diabetics either lack the hormone **insulin** entirely, or become resistant to its actions. The latter condition, which usually develops in adulthood, is termed type 2 diabetes mellitus (DM2), and accounts for 95% of diabetics. Diabetes causes progressive damage to both the microvasculature and larger arteries over many years. Approximately 75% of diabetics eventually die from CVD.

There is evidence that patients with DM2 have both endothelial damage and increased levels of oxidized LDL. Both effects may be a result of mechanisms associated with the hyperglycaemia characteristic of this condition. Also, blood coagulability is increased in DM2 because of elevated plasminogen activator inhibitor 1 (PAI-1) and increased platelet aggregability.

A set of cardiovascular risk factors including high plasma triglycerides, low plasma HDL, hypertension, elevated plasma glucose and obesity (particularly abdominal) are often associated with each other. This combination of risk factors is closely linked to, and could arise as a result of, **insulin resistance**. Individuals with three or more of these risk factors are said to have **metabolic syndrome**.

Atherosclerosis can be viewed as a chronic low-grade inflammation which is localized to certain sites of the vascular wall. This causes the release into the plasma of numerous inflammatory mediators and related substances. Many studies have shown that an elevated serum level of one of these, the acute phase reactant **C-reactive protein (CRP)**, is *predictive* of future CVD, although recent epidemiological studies, which have taken advantage of the fact that differences in the basal levels of serum CRP occur naturally in the population due to genetic variation, show that CRP does not *cause* CVD. Although proposed to be a potentially valuable risk marker that could be used to predict future CVD (and therefore indicate the need for preventative treatment) even in apparently healthy people with low LDL, many question whether

CRP levels are truly independent of other established risk factors (e.g. metabolic syndrome).

Tobacco smoking causes CVD by lowering HDL, increasing blood coagulability and damaging the endothelium, thereby promoting atherosclerosis. In addition, nicotine-induced cardiac stimulation and a carbon monoxide-mediated reduction of the oxygen-carrying capacity of the blood also occur. These effects, coupled with an increased occurrence of coronary spasm, set the stage for cardiac ischaemia and MI. Epidemiological evidence suggests that CVD risk is not reduced with low tar cigarettes.

High plasma levels of **homocysteine**, a metabolite of the amino acid methionine, are proposed to be a CVD risk factor, although the evidence for this association is controversial. Hyperhomocysteinaemia may increase cardiovascular risk by causing overproduction of the endogenous endothelial nitric oxide synthase (eNOS) inhibitor asymmetrical dimethyl arginine (**ADMA;** see Chapter 24), because homocysteine can serve as a donor of methyl groups that are enzymatically transferred to arginine to form ADMA.

Epidemiological studies show that **psychosocial stress** (e.g. depression, anxiety, anger) can substantially increase the risk of the development and recurrence of CVD. For example, the INTERHEART study reported in 2004 that people who had had an MI were more than 2.5 times as likely to report pre-existing psychosocial stress than age-matched controls. Although the reasons for this have not been definitively established, it is known that negative emotions can result in activation of the sympathetic nervous system (which can cause various deleterious effects on the cardiovascular system including a raised blood pressure and more frequent cardiac arrhythmias), and also that anxiety and depression engender unhealthy lifestyles. This may be of great importance for CVD management; one meta-analysis of 23 clinical trials reported that patients who had an MI were more than 40% less likely to die or have another MI over the next 2 years when given interventions designed to reduce psychosocial stress.

Fixed risk factors
Family history of CVD
Numerous epidemiological surveys have shown the existence of a familial predisposition to CVD. This arises in part because many CVD risk factors (e.g. hypertension) have a *multifactorial genetic basis* (are due to multiple abnormal genes interacting with environmental influences). Additional deleterious genetic influences are also probably involved, because the familial predisposition remains if epidemiological data are corrected for known risk factors. For example, the angiotensin-converting enzyme (ACE) gene can exist in two forms, characterized by the insertion or deletion of a 287-base-pair DNA segment within intron 16. Those homozygous for the deletion polymorphism have higher plasma ACE concentrations, which may modestly increase the risk of MI.

Male sex
Middle-aged women are much less likely than men to develop CVD. This difference progressively narrows after the menopause, and is mainly oestrogen mediated. The potentially beneficial actions of oestrogen include acting as an antioxidant, lowering LDL and raising HDL, stimulating the expression and activity of nitric oxide synthase, causing vasodilatation and increasing the production of plasminogen.

β-Blockers, angiotensin-converting enzyme inhibitors, angiotensin receptor blockers and Ca²⁺ channel blockers

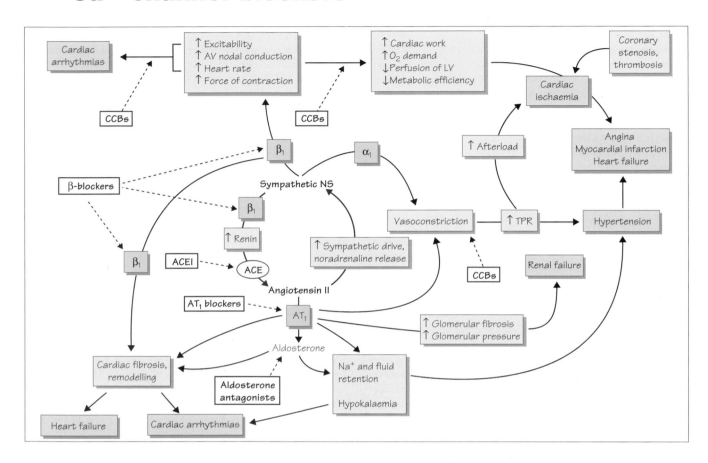

The four classes of drugs described in this chapter each stand out as being useful in treating multiple disorders of the cardiovascular system. Core aspects of their mechanisms of action and properties are described here and further details on their use are presented in the chapters dealing specifically with the disorder.

β-Adrenoceptor antagonists (β-blockers)

β-Blockers are used to treat angina, cardiac arrhythmias, myocardial infarction and chronic heart failure. Once a first line treatment for hypertension, they are now used only in combination with other antihypertensive drugs if these fail to lower blood pressure sufficiently. Their usefulness derives mainly from their blockade of cardiac β_1-receptors (Figure 35). When stimulated by noradrenaline released from sympathetic nerves, and by blood-borne adrenaline, these receptors increase the rate and force of cardiac contraction, thereby increasing the output, work and O_2 requirement of the heart. Although these responses are important for the normal physiological response to stress, they have the undesirable effect of promoting cardiac ischaemia and its downstream effects if coronary blood flow is compromised by atherosclerotic stenosis or thrombosis (see Chapters 40 and 45). Activation of β_1-receptors

also increases atrioventricular (AV) nodal conduction and the excitability of the heart, effects that can sometimes cause or promote cardiac arrhythmias (see Chapters 48 and 51). Chronic activation of the sympathetic system, as in congestive heart failure, causes cardiac fibrosis and remodelling, leading to a progressive deterioration of cardiac function and increasing the occurrence of life-threatening arrhythmias (see Chapters 46 and 48).

β-Blockers have additional useful effects. Importantly, renal afferent arterioles contain *renin-producing granular cells* which are stimulated by sympathetic nerves to release renin via their β_1-receptors. Thus, the renin–angiotensin–aldosterone (RAA) axis (see Chapter 29) can be stimulated by the sympathetic system, an effect that β-blockers inhibit. β-Blockers also decrease the release of noadrenaline from sympathetic nerves by inhibiting presynaptic β-receptors on sympathetic varicosities that act to facilitate its release.

Propranolol, a 'first generation' β-blocker, acts on both β_1 and β_2-receptors, whereas second generation β-blockers (e.g. **atenolol, metoprolol, bisoprolol**) selectively antagonize β_1-receptors. Third generation β-blockers also cause vasodilatation; for example, **carvidelol** does this by blocking α-receptors and by releasing nitric

The Cardiovascular System at a Glance, Fourth Edition. Philip I. Aaronson, Jeremy P.T. Ward, and Michelle J. Connolly.

oxide. **Pindolol** belongs to a fourth group of β-blockers with *intrinsic sympathomimetic activity*; it antagonizes β_1-receptors but stimulates β_2-receptors, thereby causing vasodilatation. Although in all cases the main therapeutic effect of these drugs lies in their effect on β_1-receptors, these various properties, as well as differences between β-blockers with respect to their pharmacokinetics and adverse effects (see below) mean that specific β-blockers may be more or less appropriate for individual patients. Adverse effects of β-blockers as a class include exercise intolerance, as well as excessive bradycardia and negative inotropy, all due to their cardiosuppressive effects. Their block of vascular β-receptors, which promote blood flow to skeletal muscle by causing vasodilatation, can also cause fatigue and cold or tingling extremities. β-Blockers also can cause bronchospasm, and are contraindicated in asthma. These drugs can also have the potentially dangerous effect of masking the perception of hypoglycaemia in diabetics.

Angiotensin-converting enzyme inhibitors and angiotensin II receptor blockers

The RAA system, acting through its effectors angiotensin II and aldosterone, has a crucial role in conserving body Na^+ and fluid, thereby acting to maintain blood volume and pressure (see Chapter 29). However, even this normal functioning of the RAA system contributes to raised blood pressure in many hypertensives (see Chapter 39), and abnormal activation of this system in those with heart failure (see Chapter 46) leads to additional adverse effects shown in the lower part of Figure 35. Angiotensin II also enhances sympathetic neurotransmission by promoting noradrenaline release and by stimulating the CNS to increase sympathetic drive, leading to further increases in blood pressure. The activity of angiotensin II can be suppressed either with angiotensin-converting enzyme inhibitors (ACEI), which block its synthesis by ACE (see Chapter 29), or by angiotensin II receptor blockers (ARBs) that inhibit its action at AT1 receptors, which mediate its various deleterious effects.

Because both block RAA system function, ACEI and ARBs suppress the various vasoconstricting effects of angiotensin II on the vasculature, thereby reducing total peripheral resistance and blood pressure. Both also cause natriuresis and diuresis which contribute to their blood pressure lowering effects and also help to reverse the pulmonary and systemic oedema and cardiac remodelling which contribute to the symptoms and progression of chronic heart failure. ACEI have the additional effect of preventing the breakdown of the peptide **bradykinin**, which is synthesized in the plasma by ACE and causes vasodilatation by releasing nitric oxide, prostacyclin and endothelium-derived hyperpolarizing factor (EDHF) from the endothelium. Increases in bradykinin may contribute to the ability of ACEI to reduce blood pressure and possibly to prevent cardiac remodelling, but may also cause the chronic cough that ACEI evoke in ~10% of people. ARBs differ from ACEI in that they do not increase bradykinin, and also in that they may cause a greater functional suppression of the RAA system because ACEI do not block *chymase*, another enzyme that synthesizes angiotensin II. Excepting the fact that ARBs cause less cough than do ACEI, the extent to which these mechanistic differences between the two types of drug are therapeutically relevant remains to be fully elucidated. At present, both ACEI and ARBs are used to treat hypertension, heart failure, myocardial infarction, and to protect against renal complications in diabetes.

The vast majority of ACEI (e.g. **enalopril**, **ramopril**, **trandolapril**; Class II) are taken orally as inactive *prodrugs* which, being lipophilic, are processed in the liver to produce an active metabolite (e.g. enalopril yields *enaloprilat*). **Captopril** (Class 1), the oldest ACEI, is itself active, but is also acted on by the liver to give active metabolites. **Lisinopril** (Class III) is active and, being water soluble, is excreted by the kidneys rather than being metabolized in the liver. Examples of ARBs include **losartan** and **candesartan**. Apart from cough, ACEI and ARBs share common contraindications and side effects. They should not be used by pregnant women because they retard fetal growth, or by those with bilateral renal stenosis, because in these individuals decreased renal blood flow typically leads to a powerful activation of the RAA system which is crucial for maintaining glomerular filtration. Because they diminish levels of aldosterone, which promotes renal K^+ excretion, both also can elevate the plasma K^+ concentration (hyperkalaemia).

Ca^{2+} channel blockers

Ca^{2+} channel blockers (CCBs) inhibit the influx of Ca^{2+} into cells through L-type Ca^{2+} channels. The interaction of blocker and Ca^{2+} channel is best understood for the *dihydropyridines* (DHPs), which include **nifedipine**, **amlodipine** and **felodipine**. The affinity of DHPs for the channel increases enormously when the channel is in its *inactivated* state (see Chapter 10). Channel inactivation is favoured by a less negative membrane potential (E_m). DHPs therefore have a relatively selective effect on vascular muscle ($E_m \sim -50$) compared with cardiac muscle ($E_m \sim -90$). This functional selectivity is further enhanced because DHP-mediated vasodilatation stimulates the baroreceptor reflex and increases sympathetic drive, overcoming any direct negative inotropic effects of these drugs. If rapid, such sympathetic activation is thought to lead to cardiac ischaemia and unstable angina, and therefore the DHPs in current use have a slow onset and prolonged effect.

The phenylalkylamine **verapamil** interacts preferentially with the channel in its *open* state. Verapamil binding is therefore less dependent on E_m; thus both cardiac and vascular Ca^{2+} channels are blocked. In addition to its vasodilating properties, verapamil therefore has negative inotropic effects and severely depresses AV nodal conduction. The benzothiazepine **diltiazem** has similar properties; at therapeutic doses it vasodilates but also depresses AV conduction and has negative inotropic/chronotropic effects.

The DHPs are currently first line agents for treating hypertension (see Chapter 38) and also all forms of angina pectoris (see Chapters 40 and 41). The non-DHPs (verapamil and diltiazem) are also used for these conditions, and are additionally used for *supraventricular cardiac arrhythmias*, based on their ability to suppress AV nodal conduction (see Chapters 49 and 51). Adverse effects of the DHPs are due to their profound vasodilating properties, and include headache, flushing and oedema. The non-DHPs can cause powerful negative inotropic and chronotropic effects, and verapamil can cause constipation.

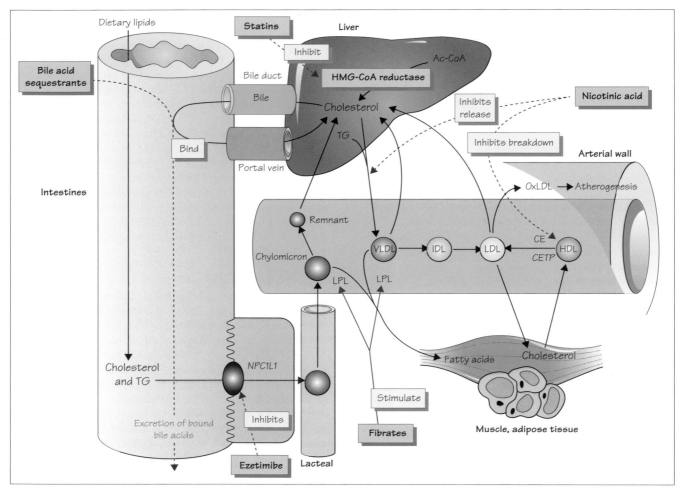

All cells require **lipids** (fats) to synthesize membranes and provide energy. Lipids are transported in the blood as **lipoproteins**. These small particles consist of a core of **triglycerides** and **cholesteryl esters**, surrounded by a coat of **phospholipids**, **cholesterol** and proteins termed **apolipoproteins** or **apoproteins**. Apoproteins stabilize the lipoprotein particles and help target specific types of lipoproteins to various tissues. **Hyperlipidaemias** are abnormalities of lipoprotein levels which promote the development of **atherosclerosis** (see Chapter 37) and coronary heart disease (CHD; see Chapters 40–42).

Lipoproteins and lipid transport

Figure 36 illustrates pathways of lipid transport in the body. The **exogenous** pathway (left side of Figure 36) delivers ingested lipids to the body tissues and liver. Ingested triglycerides and cholesterol are transported by the protein Niemann–Pick C1-like 1 (NPC1L1) into the mucosal cells lining the intestinal lumen, which combine them with apoprotein **apo B-48,** forming **nascent chylomicrons** which are secreted into the lymph, pass into the bloodstream, and combine with apo E and apo C-II to become **chylomicrons**. These bind to the capillary endothelium in muscle and adipose tissue, where apo CII activates the endothelium-bound enzyme **lipoprotein lipase** (LPL)

which hydrolyses the triglycerides to fatty acids which enter the tissues. The liver takes up the residual **chylomicron remnants**. These are broken down to yield cholesterol, which the liver also synthesizes. The rate-limiting enzyme in hepatic cholesterol synthesis is **hydroxy-methylglutaryl coenzyme A reductase** (HMG-CoA reductase). The liver uses cholesterol to make **bile acids.** These pass into the intestine and act to solubilize dietary cholesterol so it can be absorbed via NPC1L1. Bile acids are almost entirely reabsorbed and returned to the liver, although about 0.5 g/day is lost in the faeces, providing a path by which the body excretes cholesterol.

The **endogenous** pathway cycles lipids between the liver and peripheral tissues. The liver forms and secretes nascent **very low density lipoproteins** (VLDLs), consisting mainly of triglycerides with some cholesterol and apo B-100, into the lacteal vessels. These acquire apo E and apo C-II from HDL in the plasma to become VLDL. As with chylomicrons, apo C-II activates LPL causing VLDL triglyceride hydrolysis and provision of fatty acids to body tissues. As it is progressively drained of triglycerides, VLDL becomes **intermediate density lipoprotein** (IDL) and then **low-density lipoprotein** (LDL), losing all of its apoproteins (to HDL) except for **apo B-100** in the process. Most of the LDL, which contains mainly cholesteryl esters (CE), is taken up by the liver;

The Cardiovascular System at a Glance, Fourth Edition. Philip I. Aaronson, Jeremy P.T. Ward, and Michelle J. Connolly.

the rest serves to distribute cholesterol to the peripheral tissues. Cells regulate their cholesterol uptake by expressing more LDL receptors (which bind to apo B-100) when their cholesterol requirement increases.

Cholesterol is removed from tissues by **high-density lipoprotein** (HDL). HDL is initially assembled in the plasma from lipids and apoproteins (mainly **apo A1,** but also apo C-II and apo E) lost by other lipoproteins, and then progressively accumulates cholesterol (which it stores as CE) from body tissues. **Cholesteryl ester transfer protein** (CETP), which is in the plasma, transfers these from HDL to VLDL, IDL and LDL, which return them to the liver. This process by which HDL transports cholesterol to the liver from the rest of the body is termed **reverse cholesterol transport**, and probably explains why plasma HDL levels are inversely proportional to the risk of developing CHD.

Hyperlipidaemias: types and treatments

Primary hyperlipidaemias are caused by genetic abnormalities affecting apoproteins, apoprotein receptors or enzymes involved in lipoprotein metabolism, and occur in about 1 in 500 people. **Secondary hyperlipidaemias** are caused by conditions or drugs (e.g. diabetes, renal disease, alcohol abuse, thiazide diuretics) affecting lipoprotein metabolism. However, hypercholesterolaemia is most commonly caused by consumption of a diet high in saturated fats, probably because this decreases hepatic lipoprotein clearance. Although hyperlipidaemia often involves simply an excess of LDL cholesterol (LDL-C), many people, especially those with *metabolic syndrome* (see Chapter 34) have a combination of high LDL-C, high triglycerides (high VLDL), and low HDL cholesterol (HDL-C) levels in their plasma. This pattern is thought to confer a particularly large risk of developing CHD.

The treatment of hyperlipidaemias aims to slow or reverse the progression of atherosclerotic lesions by lowering LDL-C and/or triglycerides and to raise HDL-C. Current US guidelines state that LDL-C should be <160 mg/dL (4.1 mmol/L) for those who are otherwise at low risk of developing CHD, whereas for high-risk patients with existing CHD, diabetes or a 10-year risk of developing CHD of >20%, LDL-C should be <100 mg/dL (2.6 mmol/L), and ideally less than 70 mg/dL (1.8 mmol/L).

Treatment often begins with a low fat, high carbohydrate diet. If this fails to normalize hyperlipidaemia adequately after 3 months, therapy with a lipid-lowering drug is considered. The vast majority of those with high LDL-C receive 'statins', which have been consistently shown to reduce CHD and the mortality it causes. Those with high triglycerides and low HDL-C are also often given 'fibrates' or niacin (each used by ~10% of patients).

HMG-CoA reductase inhibitors or 'statins' include **simvastatin, lovastatin, pravastatin, fluvastatin, mevastatin, atorvastatin** and **rosuvastatin**. The landmark **Scandinavian Simvastatin Survival Study** (4S) reported in 1994 that treatment with simvastatin of CHD patients with high LDL-C reduced cardiovascular mortality by 42% over a 6-year period. Statins act by reducing hepatic synthesis of cholesterol, causing an upregulation of hepatic receptors for B and E apoproteins. This increases the clearance of LDL, IDL and VLDL from the plasma. Statins also modestly increase plasma HDL-C levels by an unknown mechanism. Although the main benefits of statins result from their lipid-lowering effects, they also probably reduce CHD through additional mechanisms. These include an enhancement of nitric oxide release, possibly due to

activation of the PI3K–Akt pathway (see Chapter 24), and also anti-inflammatory and antithrombotic effects. Some of these effects occur because the inhibition of HMG-CoA reduces cellular concentrations of lipids required for the functioning of the monomeric G proteins Rho (Rho acts to suppress eNOS expression) and Ras (Ras stimulates NFκB, which is involved in the expression of many pro-inflammatory genes). Serious statin-associated adverse effects are rare. They include hepatoxicity and rhabdomyolysis (destruction of skeletal muscle), the risk of which is increased with concomitant use of nicotinic acid or a fibric acid derivative.

Both **niacin (nicotinic acid)** and **fibrates (fibric acid derivatives)** are mainly used in patients who are receiving statins but whose triglyceride levels are too high (≥1.7 mmol/L or 150 mg/dL) and HDL-C levels are too low (<1.0 mmol/L or 40 mg/dL). Niacin is a B vitamin that has lipid-lowering effects at high doses. It inhibits the synthesis and release of VLDL by the liver. Because VLDL gives rise to IDL and LDL, plasma levels of these lipoproteins also fall. Conversely, HDL levels rise significantly as a result of decreased breakdown, an effect which the ARBITER 2 study (2004) showed may slow the progression of atherosclerotic plaque in patients with low HDL. Most patients experience flushing with niacin therapy. This is due to vasodilatation caused by prostaglandin release from the endothelium, and can be prevented by nonsteroidal anti-inflammatory drugs. Other reported adverse effects include hepatotoxicity, palpitations, impaired glucose tolerance, hyperuricaemia, hypotension and amblyopia.

Fibrates include **gemfibrozil, clofibrate, bezafibrate, ciprofibrate** and **fenofibrate**. Fibrates bind to peroxisome proliferator-activated receptor alpha (PPARα) to stimulate the expression and activity of LPL, thereby reducing VLDL triglycerides by increasing their hydrolysis. They also promote changes in LDL composition, which render it less atherogenic, and enhance fibrolysis. They cause mild gastrointestinal disorders in 5–10% of patients, and can potentially cause muscle toxicity and renal failure if combined with HMG-CoA reductase inhibitors or excessive alcohol use.

Bile acid sequestrants: bile acids are synthesized from cholesterol in the liver, and cycle between the liver and intestine (enterohepatic recirculation). **Cholestyramine** and **cholestipol** are exchange resins that bind and trap bile acids in the intestine, increasing their excretion. This enhances hepatic bile acid synthesis and cholesterol utilization. The resulting depletion of hepatic cholesterol causes an upregulation of LDL receptors, increasing the clearance of LDL-C from the plasma. Bile acid sequestrants cause little systemic toxicity because they are not absorbed. However, they must be taken in large amounts (up to 30 g/day) and cause gastrointestinal side effects such as emesis, diarrhoea and reflux oesophagitis, so are rarely used.

Ezetimibe reduces absorption of dietary cholesterol by inhibiting the functioning of NPC1L1. This reduces the plasma concentration and hepatic uptake of chylomicrons. The liver responds to this by expressing more LDL receptors to maintain its cholesterol uptake, and plasma LDL-C levels fall by ~15%. Ezetimibe, widely used together with statins, is a controversial drug, as the ENHANCE (2008) and ARBITER 6 (2009) studies showed that this combination was no better than a statin alone in reducing plaque progression, whereas a statin–niacin combination was.

Anacetrapib simultaneously lowers plasma LDL-C and strongly increases HDL-C by inhibiting CETP, and is currently in Phase 3 trials for treatment of atherosclerosis.

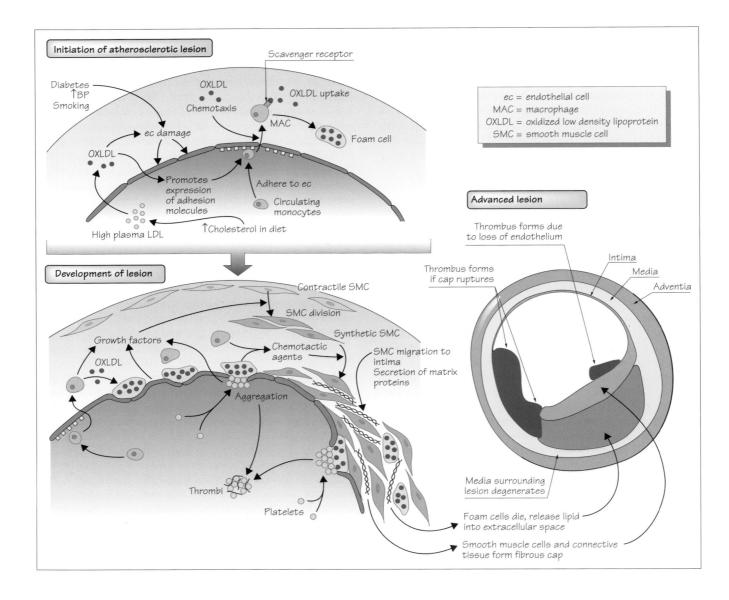

Initiation of atherosclerotic lesion

Diabetes
↑BP
Smoking

OXLDL
Chemotaxis

Scavenger receptor

OXLDL uptake

ec damage

MAC

Foam cell

OXLDL

Promotes
expression
of adhesion
molecules

Adhere to ec

Circulating
monocytes

High plasma LDL

↑Cholesterol in diet

ec = endothelial cell
MAC = macrophage
OXLDL = oxidized low density lipoprotein
SMC = smooth muscle cell

Development of lesion

Contractile SMC

SMC division

Synthetic SMC

Growth factors

Chemotactic
agents

OXLDL

SMC migration to
intima
Secretion of matrix
proteins

Aggregation

Thrombi

Platelets

Advanced lesion

Thrombus forms due
to loss of endothelium

Thrombus forms
if cap ruptures

Intima

Media

Adventia

Media surrounding
lesion degenerates

Foam cells die, release lipid
into extracellular space

Smooth muscle cells and connective
tissue form fibrous cap

Atherosclerosis is a disease of the larger arteries. It begins in childhood with localized accumulations of lipid within the arterial intima, termed **fatty streaks**. By middle age some of these develop into **atherosclerotic plaques**, focal lesions where the arterial wall is grossly abnormal. Plaques may be several centimetres across, and are most common in the *aorta*, the *coronary* and *internal carotid arteries*, and the *circle of Willis*. An advanced atherosclerotic plaque, illustrated on the right of Figure 37, demonstrates several features.

1 The arterial wall is focally thickened by intimal smooth muscle cell proliferation and the deposition of fibrous connective tissue, forming a hard **fibrous cap**. This projects into the vascular lumen,

restricting the flow of blood, and often causes ischaemia in the tissue region served by the artery.

2 A soft pool of extracellular lipid and cell debris accumulates beneath the fibrous cap (*athera* is Greek for 'gruel' or 'porridge'). This weakens the arterial wall, so that the fibrous cap may fissure or tear away. As a result, blood enters the lesions and **thrombi** (blood clots) are formed. These thrombi, or the material leaking from the ruptured lesion, may be carried to the upstream vascular bed to *embolize* (plug) smaller vessels. A larger thrombus may totally occlude (block) the artery at the site of the lesion. This causes myocardial infarction or stroke if it occurs in a coronary or cerebral artery, respectively.

The Cardiovascular System at a Glance, Fourth Edition. Philip I. Aaronson, Jeremy P.T. Ward, and Michelle J. Connolly.

3 The endothelium over the lesion is partially or completely lost. This can lead to ongoing formation of thrombi, causing intermittent flow occlusion as in unstable angina.

4 The medial smooth muscle layer under the lesion degenerates. This weakens the vascular wall, which may distend and eventually rupture (an **aneurysm**). Aneurysms are especially common in the abdominal aorta.

Atherosclerotic arteries may also demonstrate spasms or reduced vasodilatation. This worsens the restriction of the blood flow and promotes thrombus formation (see Chapters 42 and 44).

Pathogenesis of atherosclerosis

The risk of developing atherosclerosis is in part genetically determined. The incidence of clinical consequences of atherosclerosis such as ischaemic heart disease rises with age, especially after age 40. Atherosclerosis is much more common in men than in women. This difference is probably due to a protective effect of oestrogen, and progressively disappears after menopause. Important risk factors that predispose towards atherosclerosis include smoking, hypertension, diabetes and high serum cholesterol.

The most widely accepted hypothesis for the pathogenesis of atherosclerosis proposes that it is initiated by *endothelial injury or dysfunction*. Plaques tend to develop in areas of variable haemodynamic shear stress (e.g. where arteries branch or bifurcate). The endothelium is especially vulnerable to damage at such sites, as evidenced by increased endothelial cell turnover and permeability. Endothelial dysfunction promotes the adhesion of **monocytes**, white blood cells which burrow beneath the endothelial monolayer and become **macrophages**. Macrophages normally have an important role during inflammation, the body's response to injury and infection. They do so by acting as scavenger cells to remove dead cells and foreign material, and also by subsequently releasing *cytokines* and *growth factors* to promote healing. As described below, however, macrophages in the arterial wall can be abnormally activated, causing a type of slow inflammatory reaction, which eventually results in advanced and clinically dangerous plaques.

Oxidized low-density lipoprotein, macrophages and atherogenesis

Lipoproteins transport cholesterol and other lipids in the bloodstream (see Chapter 36). Elevated levels of one type of lipoprotein, low-density lipoprotein (LDL), are associated with atherosclerosis. Native LDL is not atherogenic. However, oxidative modification of LDL by oxidants derived from macrophages and endothelial and smooth muscle cells can lead to the generation of highly atherogenic **oxidized LDL** within the vascular wall.

Oxidized LDL is thought to promote atherogenesis through several mechanisms (upper panel of Figure 37). Oxidized LDL is chemotactic for (i.e. attracts) circulating monocytes, and increases the expression of endothelial cell adhesion molecules to which

monocytes attach. The monocytes then penetrate the endothelial monolayer, lodge beneath it and mature into macrophages. Cellular uptake of native LDL is normally highly regulated. However, certain cells, including macrophages, are unable to control their uptake of oxidized LDL, which occurs via **scavenger receptors**. Once within the vascular wall, macrophages therefore accumulate large quantities of oxidized LDL, eventually becoming the cholesterol-laden **foam cells** forming the fatty streak.

As shown in the lower left of Figure 37, stimulation of macrophages and endothelial cells by oxidized LDL causes these cells to release cytokines. T lymphocytes may also enter the vascular wall and release cytokines. Additional cytokines are released by platelets aggregating on the endothelium at the site at which it has been damaged by oxidized LDL and other toxic substances released by the foam cells. The cytokines act on the vascular smooth muscle cells of the media, causing them to *migrate into the intima*, to *proliferate* and to *secrete abnormal amounts of collagen and other connective tissue proteins*. Over time, the intimal accumulation of smooth muscle cells and connective tissue forms the fibrous cap on the inner arterial wall. Underneath this, ongoing foam cell formation and deterioration forms a layer of extracellular lipid (largely cholesterol and cholesteryl esters) and cellular debris. Still-viable foam cells often localize at the edges or shoulders of the lesion. Underneath the lipid, the medial layer of smooth muscle cells is weakened and atrophied.

Clinical consequences of advanced atherosclerosis

Atherosclerotic lesions are of most clinical consequence when they occur in the coronary arteries. Lesions in which the fibrous cap becomes thick tend to cause a significant **stenosis**, or narrowing of the vascular lumen, which gradually comes to cause cardiac ischaemia, especially when myocardial oxygen demand rises. This leads to **stable** or **exertional angina** (see Chapter 39). Advanced plaques often have large areas of endothelial denudation, which serve as sites for thrombus formation. In addition, lipid- and foam-cell-rich lesions are particularly unstable and prone to tearing open. This **plaque rupture** may be favoured by the presence in the lesion of T lymphocytes, as these produce interferon-γ which inhibits matrix formation, and of macrophages, which produce proteases that degrade the connective tissue matrix. Plaque rupture allows blood to enter the lesion, causing thrombi to form on the surface and/or within the lesion, often resulting in an acute coronary syndrome such as unstable angina (see Chapter 42) or myocardial infarction (see Chapter 43). Non-fatal chronic thrombi may gradually be replaced by connective tissue and incorporated into the lesion, a process termed **organization**. Atherosclerosis of cerebral arteries is the major cause of **stroke** (cerebral infarction). Atherosclerotic stenosis of the renal arteries causes about two-thirds of cases of **renovascular hypertension**.

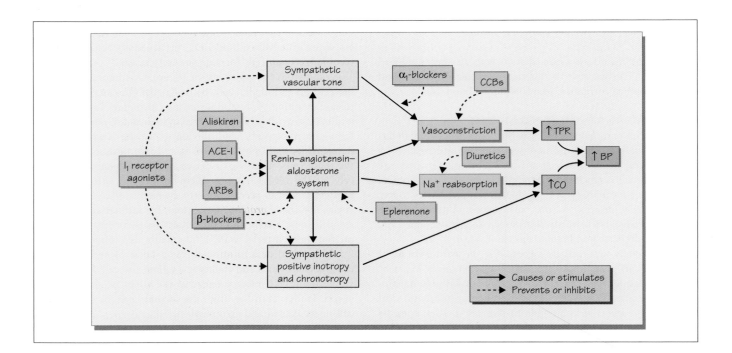

Hypertension is defined pragmatically as the level of blood pressure (BP) above which therapeutic intervention can be shown to reduce the risk of developing cardiovascular disease (Table 38.1). Risk increases progressively with *both* systolic and diastolic BP levels. Epidemiological studies predict that a long-term 5–6-mmHg diminution of diastolic blood pressure (DBP) should reduce the incidence of stroke and CHD by about 40 and 25%, respectively. However, rises in systolic pressure are now given more emphasis and **isolated systolic hypertension** (ISH), which often develops in the elderly, is particularly deleterious.

Individual BP measurements can vary significantly, and current guidelines state that, unless severe, hypertension (BP>140/90 mmHg) initially detected in the clinic should be confirmed using an ambulatory BP monitor which records multiple BP measurements over a 24-hour period. Tests for damage to target organs vulnerable to hypertension (e.g. eyes, kidneys) and assessment of other cardiovascular risk factors should also be carried out. Those with stage 1 hypertension should then be treated if they have overt cardiovascular disease, diabetes, target organ damage, renal disease or an overall cardiovascular risk of >20% per 10 years (as estimated using risk tables derived from the Framingham study; see Chapter 34). All those with stage 2 or 3 hypertension should be treated. The goal of antihypertensive therapy is to reduce the blood pressure to below 140/90 mmHg (or to below 130/80 mmHg in diabetics and those with renal disease).

Lifestyle modifications such as *weight reduction*, *regular aerobic exercise* and *limitation of dietary sodium* and *alcohol intake* can often normalize pressure in mild hypertensives. They are also useful adjuncts to pharmacological therapy of more severe disease,

Table 38.1 Classification of adult blood pressure by the US Joint National Committee on Detection, Evaluation and Treatment of High Blood Pressure. HT, hypertension.

Classification	Systolic (mmHg)		Diastolic (mmHg)
Normotension	<130	*and/or*	<85
High normal	130–139	*and/or*	85–89
Stage 1 HT	140–159	*and/or*	90–99
Stage 2 HT	160–179	*and/or*	100–109
Stage 3 HT	>180	*and/or*	>110

and have the important added bonus of reducing overall cardiovascular risk. However, adequate BP control usually requires the lifelong use of **antihypertensive drugs.** These act to reduce cardiac output and/or total peripheral resistance.

Thiazide diuretics cause an initial increased Na^+ excretion by the kidneys, which is due to inhibition of Na^+/Cl^- symport in the distal nephron. This leads to a fall in blood volume and cardiac output. Subsequently, blood volume recovers, but total peripheral resistance falls due to an unknown mechanism. Thiazide diuretics (e.g. chlorthalidone, indapamide) can cause hypokalaemia by promoting Na^+–K^+ exchange in the collecting tubule. This can be prevented by giving K^+ supplements, or also by combining thiazide diuretics with K^+-sparing diuretics (e.g. amiloride) to reduce Na^+ reabsorption and therefore K^+ secretion by blocking Na^+ channels (EnaC) in the collecting duct. Additional side effects include increases in plasma insulin, glucose or cholesterol, as well as hypersensitivity reactions and impotence.

The Cardiovascular System at a Glance, Fourth Edition. Philip I. Aaronson, Jeremy P.T. Ward, and Michelle J. Connolly.

Angiotensin-converting enzyme inhibitors (ACEI) such as **captopril**, **enalopril** and **lisinopril** block the conversion of angiotensin I into angiotensin II. This reduces total peripheral resistance because angiotensin II stimulates the sympathetic system centrally, promotes release of noradrenaline from sympathetic nerves, and vasoconstricts directly. The fall in plasma angiotensin II, and consequently in aldosterone, also promotes diuresis/natriuresis because both hormones cause renal Na^+ and water retention (see Chapter 29). ACE also metabolizes the vasodilators bradykinin and substance P, and part of the beneficial action of ACEI may be due to elevated levels of bradykinin. However, increases in bradykinin and substance P may also sensitize sensory nerves in the airways, leading to the chronic cough that is the most common adverse effect of ACEI. This effect does not occur with **angiotensin II receptor (AT_1) blockers** (ARB) such as **losartan** and **valsartan**, which selectively inhibit the effects of angiotensin II on its AT_1 subtype without affecting bradykinin levels. Both ACEI and ARB have few side effects, leading to their increasing popularity. However, they are contraindicated in pregnancy, renovascular disease and aortic stenosis. **Eplerenone**, a selective *aldosterone receptor antagonist* (see also Chapter 47), is also used to treat hypertension, as is the newer drug **aliskiren**, an antagonist of renin which prevents it from producing angiotensin I.

Calcium-channel blockers (CCBs) such as **nifedipine**, **verapamil** and **diltiazem** are commonly used to treat hypertension due to their vasodilating properties, as described in Chapter 35. The dihydropyridine CCBs, which are selective for vascular smooth muscle over the heart, are used most widely, and also have a useful diuretic effect. The 2005 ASCOT trial showed that the long-acting dihydropyridine **amlodipine** (with the ACEI perindopril added in if required to meet blood pressure targets) reduced cardiovascular morbidity and mortality more effectively than the β-blocker atenolol (with the diuretic bendroflumethiazide if required). DHPs have been shown to be especially effective in the elderly, and are safe in pregnancy.

In view of the results of ASCOT and other recent clinical trials, **β-receptor blockers** (see Chapter 35), once a first line treatment for hypertension, are now recommended for use mainly in combination with other drugs in patients who do not respond well to treatment. β-Blockers antagonize sympathetic nervous system stimulation of cardiac β-receptors (mainly $β_1$), thereby reducing cardiac output through negative inotropic and chronotropic effects. They also block β-receptors on juxtaglomerular granule cells in the kidney, thus inhibiting renin release and reducing plasma levels of angiotensin II and aldosterone. During treatment, total peripheral resistance rises initially and then returns to the predrug level via an unknown mechanism, while cardiac output remains depressed. Some β-blockers are selective for the $β_1$ subtype (atenolol), while others block both $β_1$ and $β_2$ subtypes (propranolol), and several (pindolol) are partial β-receptor agonists. In each case, the effects on blood pressure are similar, although the partial β-receptor agonists are probably acting more as vasodilators than by reducing cardiac output. All β-blockers are contraindicated in moderate/severe asthma due to their potential effects on bronchiolar $β_2$-receptors. Adverse effects of these drugs include fatigue, negative inotropy, CNS disturbances in some (e.g. nightmares), and worsening and masking of the signs of hypoglycaemia.

$α_1$-receptor-selective blockers cause vasodilatation by inhibiting the ongoing constriction of arteries by the sympathetic neurotransmitter noradrenaline. These drugs are used in preference to non-selective α-antagonists in order to prevent the increased norepinephrine release from sympathetic nerves that would occur if presynaptic $α_2$-receptors were also blocked. Like β-blockers, these drugs are used at a late stage of stepped treatment if combinations of other drugs have failed to adequately control the blood pressure.

The drugs **rilmenidine** and **moxonidine** reduce sympathetic outflow by activating central **imidazoline** (I_1) receptors in the rostral ventrolateral medulla (RVLM). This lowers blood pressure with few side effects, but the use of these drugs is limited due to the present lack of evidence from clinical trials that they have beneficial effects on survival.

Stepped treatment: treatment of hypertension is typically initiated with a single drug, but combinations of several drugs are usually needed to achieve adequate blood pressure control. The renin–angiotensin–aldosterone axis is more likely to be a contributing factor in causing hypertension in younger white patients, and so *step 1* is to try an ACEI or ARB in white patients <55 of age and a CCB or a diuretic in black and older white hypertensives. If this fails to control BP, *step 2* in all patients is to try a combination of a CCB or diuretic with an ACE-I or ARB. If BP is still not lowered enough, *step 3* is to use an (ACE-I or ARB)/CCB/diuretic combination. Antagonists to aldosterone and α- or β-receptors, or other drugs, can then be tried in *step 4*. Drug selection is also influenced by whether a patient has a coexisting condition which renders a certain type of antihypertensive more or less appropriate in that individual (e.g. ACEI are also useful for treating heart failure and diabetic nephropathy but should not be used in pregnant women; Ca^{2+} channel blockers are used to control angina).

In cases in which hypertension is secondary to a known condition or factor (e.g. renal stenosis, oral contraceptives), removal of this cause is often sufficient to normalize the blood pressure.

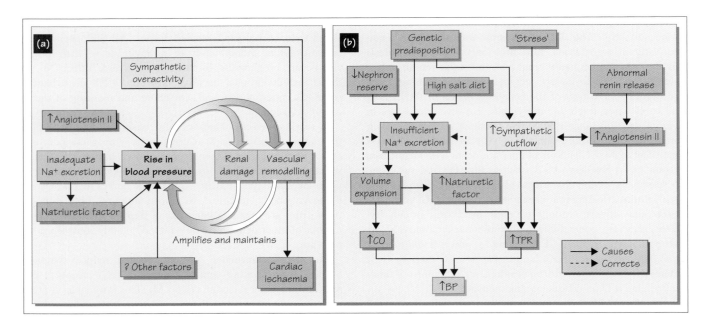

In more than 90% of cases, hypertension has no obvious cause, and is termed **primary** or **essential**. Primary hypertension is a **complex genetic disease**, in which the inheritance of a number of commonly occurring gene *alleles* (different forms of a gene that arise by mutation and code for alternative forms of a protein that may show functional differences) predisposes an individual to high arterial blood pressure (ABP), especially if appropriate *environmental influences* (e.g. high salt diet, psychosocial stress) are also present. It is thought that proteins coded for by hundreds of genes may affect blood pressure, with the allelic variation of each causing only a small effect on blood pressure. Given this genetic complexity, investigations into the mechanisms causing high blood pressure have mainly focused on uncovering functional rather than genetic abnormalities, often using strains of animals that are selectively bred to develop high ABP in the hope that the mechanisms causing hypertension in these are similar to those in humans. However, the recent advent of large genome-wide association studies has now begun to allow the tentative identification of genes having alternative alleles that affect blood pressure; one of these is *ATP2B1*, the gene coding for the plasma membrane Ca^{2+} ATPase (see Chapter 15).

Studies tracking cardiovascular function over decades show that human hypertension is initially associated with an increased cardiac output (CO) and heart rate, but a normal total peripheral resistance (TPR). Over a period of years, CO falls to subnormal levels, while TPR becomes permanently increased, thereby maintaining the hypertension (recall that $ABP = CO \times TPR$). These observations imply that the factors maintaining high ABP change over time. Therefore the mechanisms that initiate high ABP (e.g. insufficient Na^+ excretion, sympathetic overactivity) may then be succeeded and/or amplified by additional common secondary mechanisms (e.g. renal damage and vascular structural remodelling) which are caused by, and maintain, the initial rise in pressure. This unifying hypothesis for primary hypertension is shown in Figure 39a.

The kidney and sodium in hypertension

Guyton's model of hypertension The kidneys regulate long-term ABP by controlling the body's Na^+ content (see Chapter 29). Guyton proposed that hypertension is initiated by renal abnormalities which cause *impaired* or *inadequate Na^+ excretion* (Figure 39b). The resulting Na^+ retention increases blood volume, and therefore CO and ABP. These changes then promote Na^+ excretion by causing **pressure natriuresis** (see Chapter 29). Fluid balance is therefore restored, but at the cost of a rise in ABP. Guyton further hypothesized that the rise in ABP or flow sets in train autoregulatory processes resulting in long-term vasoconstriction and/or vascular structural remodelling. This would reduce blood volume to normal levels, but by raising TPR would maintain the high ABP needed for Na^+ balance.

There is extensive evidence that a renal mechanism of hypertension is important in many people. For example, a high salt diet, which should exacerbate the renal deficiency in Na^+ excretion, worsens hypertension in many patients and, as shown in the Intersalt study, seems to cause a slow rise in ABP over many years in most people. It has also been shown that ABP falls when the kidneys from normotensives are transplanted into hypertensives. Moreover, hypertension occurs in **Liddle syndrome**, a condition in which a mutation of the mineralocorticoid-sensitive Na^+ channel (ENaC) impairs renal Na^+ excretion.

The natriuretic factor hypothesis De Wardener and others have proposed that the body responds to inadequate renal salt excretion by producing one or more **natriuretic factors** (not to be confused with **atrial natriuretic peptide**; see Chapter 29) which promote salt excretion by inhibiting the Na^+–K^+-ATPase in the nephron. Although this effect would be expected to reduce ABP, the Na^+–K^+-ATPase is also indirectly involved in lowering intracellular Ca^{2+}, via regulation of both the membrane potential and Na^+–Ca^{2+} exchange, in smooth muscle cells and neurones. Natriuretic factors

The Cardiovascular System at a Glance, Fourth Edition. Philip I. Aaronson, Jeremy P.T. Ward, and Michelle J. Connolly.

would therefore cause additional responses such as vasoconstriction, increased noradrenaline release, and possibly stimulation of brain centres involved in raising ABP. These effects would increase TPR, causing sustained hypertension. In agreement with this hypothesis, **ouabain-like factor** and **marinobufagenin**, two endogenous substances that inhibit the Na^+–K^+-ATPase, are elevated in plasma taken from many hypertensives.

The reduced nephron number hypothesis Brenner and coworkers have proposed that many hypertensives have a congenital reduction in the number, or filtering ability, of their nephrons which would cause the inadequate Na^+ excretion referred to above. Evidence suggests that this may arise from intrauterine growth retardation.

Neurogenic and humoral theories of hypertension

A considerable body of evidence supports the concept that an overactivity of the renin–angiotensin–aldosterone (RAA) system, which has a crucial role in regulating renal Na^+ excretion, occurs in many hypertensives, and is responsible for the defect in renal Na^+ excretion originally proposed by Guyton. Although renin release should be greatly suppressed by elevated ABP (as explained in Chapter 29), ~70% of hypertensives have normal or high plasma renin activity, suggesting that their RAA system is inappropriately activated. This would cause Na^+ retention due to increased effects of angiotensin II and aldosterone in the kidney (see Chapter 29), and also lead to angiotensin II-mediated vasoconstriction throughout the body. Both mechanisms would raise ABP. Primary hypertension in some individuals has also been linked to a mutation in the **angiotensinogen** gene, which could promote increased angiotensin II production. Most importantly, drugs that inhibit this system effectively control ABP in ~50% of hypertensive individuals (see Chapter 38). Interestingly, the kidney is now thought to have its own renin–angiotensin system which is regulated independently of the RAA system in the rest of the body. Recent studies with mice in which the AT_1 receptor was knocked out only in the kidney suggest that it is this 'intra-renal' renin–angiotensin system that may be of predominant importance in causing hypertension, although whether this is also true in humans is unknown.

The **neurogenic model of hypertension** proposes that hypertension is primarily initiated by overactivity of the sympathetic nervous system. Although the kidneys are central to controlling ABP, supporters of this concept argue that the kidneys (and in particular renin release) are themselves regulated by the sympathetic nervous system, which therefore must be the ultimate determinant of ABP. The neurogenic model is supported by evidence that sympathetic nervous activity is increased in young borderline hypertensives, by the fact that drugs such as moxonidine, which act in the brain to reduce sympathetic outflow, effectively lower ABP (see Chapter 38), and by the results of the Simplicity HTN-2 trial, which reported in 2010 that renal sympathetic denervation caused a sustained fall in blood pressure in a group of 'resistant' hypertensives whose blood pressure could not be controlled pharmacologically. Sympathetic overactivity is thought to occur in ~50% of hypertensives, and could potentially be caused by a variety of factors that have been shown to stimulate areas of the brainstem that control sympathetic outflow; these include inflammation, hypoxia, elevated reactive oxygen species or overactivity of the RAA system.

Insulin resistance is a condition in which the body becomes less responsive to the actions of the hormone *insulin*, leading to a compensatory rise in plasma insulin levels. Both insulin resistance and obesity, with which it is often associated, are very common in hypertensives. There is evidence that excessive insulin can cause multiple effects on the body which could promote hypertension, including activation of the sympathetic nervous system, increased renal Na^+ reabsorption and reduced endothelium-dependent vasodilatation.

Vascular remodelling

Established hypertension is associated with the *structural alteration* of small arteries and larger arterioles. This process, termed **remodelling**, results in the narrowing of these vessels and an increase in the ratio of wall thickness to luminal radius. Remodelling is proposed to be an adaptive mechanism which would reduce vascular wall stress (see the Laplace/Frank law; see Chapter 18) and protect the microcirculation from increased ABP. However, it would also 'lock in' vascular narrowing and the resulting increase in TPR. Remodelling may also be enhanced by overactivation of the RAA and sympathetic nervous systems, which is known to promote smooth muscle cell growth.

Remodelling will increase basal TPR and also exaggerate any increase in TPR caused by vasoconstriction. In addition, studies in *spontaneously hypertensive rats* indicate that remodelling of renal afferent arterioles may contribute to hypertension by interfering with renal Na^+ excretion (see above). This implies that remodelling would accentuate increases in ABP caused by other factors, thereby contributing to the vicious cycle illustrated in Figure 39a. In addition, remodelling of the coronary arteries as a result of hypertension may increase the risk of myocardial infarction by restricting the ability of these vessels to increase the cardiac blood supply during ischaemia.

Secondary hypertension

In less than 10% of cases, high ABP is secondary to a known condition or factor. Common causes of **secondary hypertension** include:

1 *Renal parenchymal* and *renovascular diseases*, which impair volume regulation and/or activate the RAA system
2 *Endocrine disturbances*, often of the adrenal cortex, and associated with oversecretion of aldosterone, cortisol and/or catecholamines
3 *Oral contraceptives*, which may raise ABP via RAA activation and hyperinsulinaemia.

Malignant or accelerated hypertension is an uncommon condition that develops quickly, involves large elevations in pressure, is often secondary to other conditions, rapidly damages the kidneys, retina, brain and heart, and if untreated causes death within 1–2 years.

Consequences of hypertension

Chronic hypertension causes changes in the arteries similar to those due to ageing. These include endothelial damage and **arteriosclerosis**, a thickening and increased connective tissue content of the arterial wall that reduces arterial compliance. These effects on vascular structure combine with elevated arterial pressure to promote atherosclerosis, coronary heart disease, left ventricular hypertrophy and renal damage. Hypertension is therefore an important risk factor for *myocardial infarction, congestive heart failure, stroke* and *renal failure*.

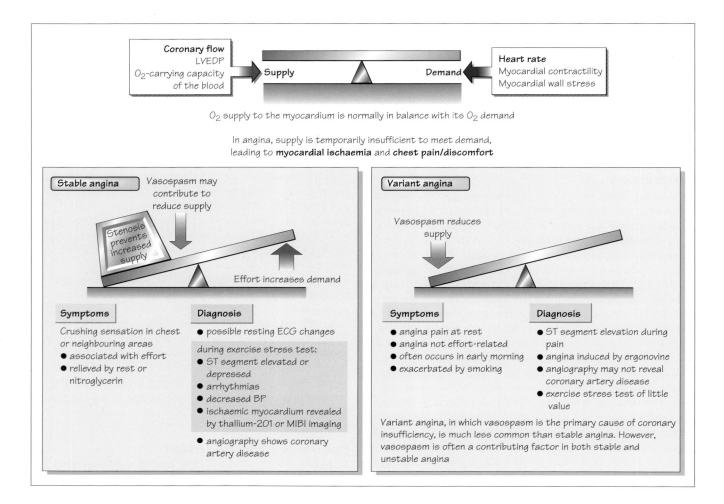

Angina pectoris is an episodic pain or crushing and/or squeezing sensation in the chest caused by reversible myocardial ischaemia. The discomfort may radiate into the neck, jaw and arms (particularly the left) and, more rarely, into the back. Other common symptoms include shortness of breath, abdominal pain and dizziness. Syncope (unconsciousness) occurs infrequently. Ischaemia can produce classic angina or may be totally *silent* without any symptoms. The clinical outlook from silent ischaemia is similar to symptomatic angina.

Three forms of angina are recognized. **Stable** and **variant** angina are discussed below, and **unstable angina** is described in Chapter 42.

Pathophysiology

Figure 40 shows the factors that determine myocardial O_2 supply and demand. O_2 demand is determined by **heart rate**, **left ventricular contractility** and **systolic wall stress**, and therefore increases with **exercise**, **hypertension** and **left ventricular dilatation** (e.g. during chronic heart failure). Myocardial O_2 supply is primarily determined by coronary blood flow and coronary vascular resistance, which mostly occurs at the level of the intramyocardial arte-

rioles. With exercise the coronary blood flow can increase to four to six times baseline, which is the normal coronary flow reserve (see Chapter 23).

Stable or **exertional (typical)** angina arises when the flow reserve of one or more coronary arteries is limited by a significant structural stenosis (>70%) resulting from atherosclerotic coronary heart disease. Stenoses typically develop in the epicardial region of arteries, within 6 cm of the aorta. Under resting conditions, cardiac O_2 demand is low enough to be satisfied even by a diminished coronary flow. However, when exertion or emotional stress increases myocardial O_2 demand, dilatation of the non-diseased areas of the artery cannot increase the supply of blood to the heart because the stenosis presents a fixed non-dilating obstruction. The resulting imbalance between myocardial O_2 demand and supply causes myocardial ischaemia. Ischaemia develops mainly in the **subendocardium**, the inner part of the myocardial wall. This is because the blood flow to the left ventricular wall occurs mainly during diastole as a result of arteriolar compression during systole. The arterioles of the subendocardium are compressed more than those of the mid- or subepicardial layers, so that the subendocardium is most vulnerable to a relative lack of O_2.

The Cardiovascular System at a Glance, Fourth Edition. Philip I. Aaronson, Jeremy P.T. Ward, and Michelle J. Connolly.

In addition to causing pain, ischaemia causes a decline in myocardial cell high-energy phosphates (creatine phosphate and ATP). As a result, both ventricular contractility and diastolic relaxation in the territory of affected arteries are impaired. Consequences of these events may include a fall in cardiac output, symptoms of pulmonary congestion and activation of the sympathetic nervous system. Stable angina is almost always relieved within 5–10 min by rest or by nitroglycerin, which reduces cardiac O_2 demand.

Some patients with stable angina may have excellent effort tolerance one day, but develop angina with minimal activity on another day. Contributing to this phenomenon of *variable threshold angina* is a dynamic endothelial dysfunction which often occurs in patients with coronary artery disease. The endothelium normally acts via nitric oxide to dilate coronary arteries during exercise. If this endothelium-dependent vasodilatation is periodically impaired, exercise may result in paradoxical vasoconstriction due to the unopposed vasoconstricting effect of the sympathetic nervous system on coronary α-receptors.

Variant angina, also termed **vasospastic** or **Prinzmetal's** angina, is an uncommon condition in which myocardial ischaemia and pain are caused by a severe transient *occlusive spasm* of one or more epicardial coronary arteries. Patients with variant angina may or may not have coronary atherosclerosis, and in the former case, vasospasm often occurs in the vicinity of plaques. Variant angina occurs at rest (typically in the early morning hours) and may be intensely painful. It is exacerbated by smoking, and can be precipitated by cocaine use. About 30% of these patients show no evidence of coronary atherosclerotic lesions. Vasospasm is thought to occur because a segment of artery becomes abnormally overreactive to vasoconstricting agents (e.g. noradrenaline, serotonin). There is also evidence that flow-mediated vasodilatation, a function of the endothelium, is impaired in the coronary arteries of patients with variant angina, and that this endothelial dysfunction may be due to oxidative stress (see Chapter 24).

Diagnosis

Ischaemic heart disease and stable angina can be distinguished from other conditions causing chest pain (e.g. neuromuscular disorders, gastroesophageal reflux) based on characteristic anginal symptoms and several types of diagnostic investigation. Although *resting ST/T wave changes* indicate severe underlying coronary artery disease, the resting ECG is often normal. In this case, the presence of ischaemic heart disease can be unmasked by an **exercise stress test**, during which patients exercise at progressively increasing levels of effort on a stationary bicycle or treadmill. Development of cardiac ischaemia is revealed by chest pain, ECG changes including *ST segment depression* or *elevation*, arrhythmias, or a fall in blood pressure due to reduced ventricular contractility. The degree of effort at which these signs develop indicates the severity of ischaemia.

The exercise stress test is less useful in uncovering ischaemia-related ECG changes if the baseline ECG is already abnormal due to factors such as left bundle branch block. In such patients, techniques designed to visualize ischaemic myocardium can be combined with the stress test to increase its specificity. **Thallium-201** is an isotope that is taken up by normal but not ischaemic or previously infarcted myocardium. It is given intravenously during the stress test, and a gamma camera is used to image its distribution in the heart both immediately and also after the test, when ischaemia has subsided. A region of exercise-induced ischaemia will cause a 'cold spot' during but not after the stress test, because it will take up thallium-201 only when ischaemia has passed. Technetium-99m (^{99m}Tc)-labelled sestamibi (see Chapter 33) can also be used for this purpose. **Coronary angiography** (see Chapter 33) is used to provide direct radiographic visualization of the extent and severity of coronary artery disease, allowing risk assessment.

The hallmark of variant angina is ST segment elevation on the ECG. Cardiac ischaemia caused by variant angina can cause ventricular arrhythmias, syncope and even myocardial infarction during prolonged attacks. Variant angina can be provoked by intravenous administration of the vasoconstrictor **ergonovine**, forming the basis of a hospital test for this condition.

Prognosis
Stable angina
Uncomplicated stable angina has a good prognosis. Epidemiological studies show that cardiovascular mortality in patients with stable angina is approximately 1% per year. Mortality increases with the number of diseased arteries, especially if there is significant stenosis in the left coronary artery mainstem. Patients who have poor left ventricular function or diabetes are also at particular risk.

Variant angina
Patients without significant coronary artery disease have a benign prognosis; in a recent study only 4% of patients in this group died from a cardiac cause during an average follow-up period of 7 years. However, patients who also have severe coronary artery disease or who develop severe arrhythmias during vasospastic episodes are at greater risk.

Management
The management of angina is designed to control symptoms, reduce underlying risk factors and improve prognosis. **Control of symptoms** involves the use of nitrovasodilators, β-adrenoceptor blockers and Ca^{2+} channel antagonists (see Chapter 41). Minimization of **risk factors** involves the use of low-dose aspirin, lipid-lowering drugs and lifestyle changes, and is a vital component of treatment. Revascularization (see Chapter 43) can also be used to treat stable angina.

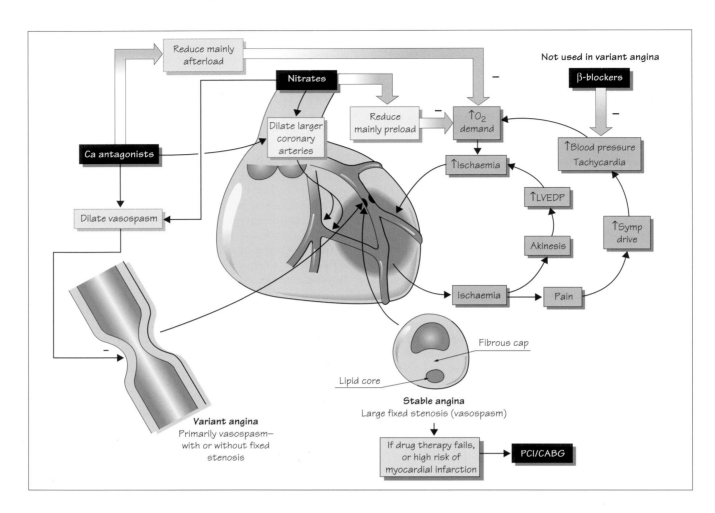

Variant angina
Primarily vasospasm—
with or without fixed
stenosis

Stable angina
Large fixed stenosis (vasospasm)

The aim of treatment of stable angina is twofold: to control symptoms and to halt the progression of underlying coronary heart disease. Anti-anginals control symptoms and work by restoring the balance between myocardial O_2 demand and supply. Patients whose stable angina is refractory to pharmacological agents should be considered for revascularization with coronary artery angioplasty or bypass grafting. The treatment of **variant angina** is primarily directed at reversing coronary **vasospasm**.

Anti-anginals

First line treatment for stable angina consists of either a β-adrenergic receptor blocker (**β-blocker**), or a **calcium-channel blocker** (CCB) together with a short-acting nitrate. If the patient's symptoms are inadequately controlled on one sole agent, and if comorbidities permit, a combination may be used. If in spite of optimal doses of both β-blocker and CCB, the patient still reports anginal pain, other drugs could be added such as ivadrabine, nicorandil, ranolazine and a long-acting nitrate. The initial choice between a β-blocker or a CCB is influenced by coexisting conditions and contraindications. For example, a CCB is preferable if the patient has moderate or severe asthma or hypertension, and a β-blocker may be the choice if rate control is also required (i.e. if atrial fibrillation is also present). If the patient cannot tolerate either of these agents, then monotherapy with a **long-acting nitro-vasodilator** should be commenced. Some patients need to take multiple classes of anti-anginal to control their symptoms.

β-Adrenergic receptor blockers

As Figure 41 illustrates, myocardial ischaemia creates a vicious cycle by activating the sympathetic nervous system and increasing ventricular end-diastolic pressure; both these effects then trigger ischaemia and anginal pain. **β-Blockers** help to block this cycle, thereby decreasing O_2 demand. They reduce O_2 demand by decreasing myocardial contractility and wall stress. The resting and exercising heart rate also falls. This increases the fraction of time the heart spends in diastole, thus enhancing perfusion of the coronary arteries, which occurs predominantly during diastole. The main

The Cardiovascular System at a Glance, Fourth Edition. Philip I. Aaronson, Jeremy P.T. Ward, and Michelle J. Connolly.

therapeutic action of these drugs is on cardiac β_1-receptors, but both β_1-selective and (β_1/β_2) non-selective blockers are used.

Potential adverse effects of β-blockers include fatigue, reduced left ventricular function and severe bradycardia. Impotence may be a concern in men. β-Blockers can precipitate asthma by blocking β_2-receptors in the airways, and therefore even β_1-selective agents are contraindicated in this condition. Lipid-soluble β-blockers (e.g. propranolol) can enter the central nervous system and cause depression or nightmares. β-Blockers can also worsen insulin-induced hypoglycaemia in diabetics.

Ca^{2+}-channel blockers (also Ca^{2+} antagonists)

CCBs act by blocking the L-type voltage-gated Ca^{2+} channels that allow depolarization-mediated influx of Ca^{2+} into smooth muscle cells, and also cardiac myocytes (see Chapters 11, 13 and 35). As described in Chapter 35, *dihydropyridine* CCBs such as **amlodipine**, **nifedipine** and **felodipine** act selectively on vascular L-type Ca^{2+} channels, while the phenylalkylamine **verapamil** and the benzothiazepine **diltiazem** block these channels in both blood vessels and the heart.

CCBs prevent angina mainly by causing systemic arteriolar vasodilatation and decreasing afterload. They also prevent coronary vasospasm, making them particularly useful in variant angina. Their use is theoretically advantageous in variable threshold angina, in which coronary vasoconstriction contributes to reduced coronary artery perfusion (see Chapter 40). The negative inotropic and chronotropic effects of verapamil and diltiazem also contribute to their usefulness by reducing myocardial O_2 demand.

The vasodilatation caused by CCBs can cause hypotension, headache and peripheral oedema (mainly dihydropyridines). On the other hand, their cardiac effects can elicit excessive cardiodepression and atrioventricular (AV) node conduction block (mainly verapamil and diltiazem). CCBs are contraindicated in acute cardiac failure. Caution is required before prescribing CCBs and β-blockers together as the combination can cause dangerous bradycardia.

Nitrovasodilators

Nitrovasodilators include **glyceryl trinitrate (GTN)**, **isosorbide mononitrate**, **isosorbide dinitrate**, **erythrityl tetranitrate** and **pentaerythritol tetranitrate**. Rapidly acting nitrovasodilators are used to terminate acute attacks of angina, while longer-acting preparations provide long-term reduction in angina symptoms.

Nitrovasodilators are metabolized to release nitric oxide (NO), thus acting as a 'pharmacological endothelium'. The mechanisms of metabolism are unclear, although nitroglycerin is thought to be metabolized mainly by the enzyme *mitochondrial aldehyde dehydrogenase*. NO stimulates guanylate cyclase to elevate cGMP, thereby causing vasodilatation (see Chapter 24). At therapeutic doses, nitrovasodilators act primarily to dilate veins, thus reducing central venous pressure (preload) and as a consequent ventricular end-diastolic volume. This lowers myocardial contraction, wall stress and O_2 demand. Some arterial dilatation also occurs, diminishing total peripheral resistance (afterload). This allows the left ventricle to maintain cardiac output with a smaller stroke volume, again decreasing O_2 demand.

Nitrovasodilators can also increase the perfusion of ischaemic myocardium. They dilate larger coronary arteries (those >100 µm in diameter). These give rise to **collateral vessels** (see Chapter 3) which can bypass stenotic arteries. Collaterals increase in number and diameter in the presence of a significant stenosis, providing an alternative perfusion of ischaemic tissue which is then enhanced by the nitrovasodilators. Nitrovasodilators also relieve coronary vasospasm, and may diminish plaque-related platelet aggregation and thrombosis by elevating platelet cGMP.

GTN taken sublingually relieves angina within minutes; this route of administration avoids the extensive first-pass metabolism of these drugs associated with oral dosing. Nitrovasodilators can also be given in slowly absorbed oral, transdermal and buccal forms for sustained effect.

Continuous exposure to nitrovasodilators causes **tolerance**. This is caused in part by increased production within blood vessels of reactive oxygen species, which may inactivate NO and also interfere with nitrovasodilator bioconversion. Reflex activation of the renin–angiotensin–aldosterone system by nitrovasodilator-induced vasodilatation may also contribute to tolerance. Tolerance is irrelevant with short-acting nitrovasodilators, but long-acting preparations become ineffective within hours. Tolerance can be minimized by 'eccentric' dosing schedules that allow blood concentrations to become low overnight. The most important adverse effect of nitrovasodilators is headache. Reflex tachycardia and orthostatic hypotension may also occur.

Other anti-anginals

Drugs used less frequently for angina include **nicorandil,** a vasodilator that has nitrate-like effects and also opens potassium channels; **ivabradine**, which reduces cardiac ischaemia by inhibiting the cardiac pacemaker current I_f (see Chapter 11) and slowing the heart; and **ranolazine**, which protects against ischaemia by increasing glucose metabolism compared to that of fatty acids.

Management of variant angina

CCBs and nitrovasodilators are also used to treat variant angina, but β-blockers are *not*, as they may worsen coronary vasospasm by blocking the β_2-mediated (vasodilating), but not α_1-mediated (vasoconstricting) effects of sympathetic stimulation.

Drugs for secondary prevention of cardiovascular disease

The reduction of risk factors that contribute to the further progression of coronary artery disease is a key aim of angina management. Patients should be treated with 75 mg/day aspirin, which suppresses platelet aggregation and greatly reduces the risk of myocardial infarction and death in patients with both stable and unstable angina. Patients should be offered a statin (e.g. 10 mg atorvastatin; see Chapter 36) to reduce their plasma LDL levels. The 2001 HOPE trial showed that the angiotensin-converting enzyme inhibitor (ACEI) ramipril reduced the progression of atherosclerosis and enhanced survival over a period of 5 years, in a group with coronary artery disease or diabetes, and ACEI are recommended for patients with stable angina who also have other conditions (e.g. hypertension or heart failure) for which these drugs are indicated.

42 Acute coronary syndromes: Unstable angina and non-ST segment elevation myocardial infarction

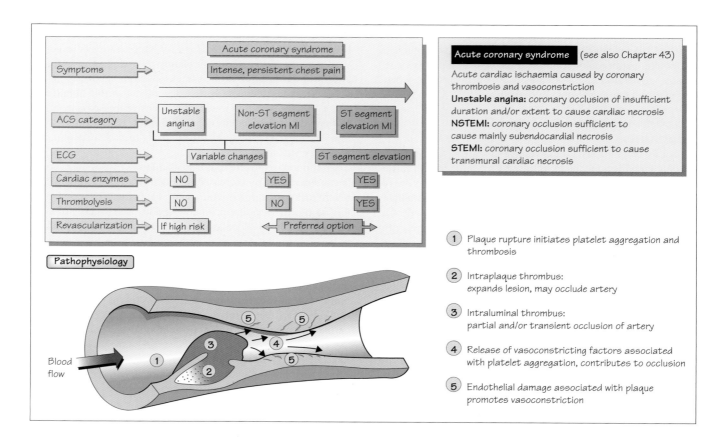

Stable angina is a chronic condition that occurs on a relatively predictable basis on exertion when cardiac ischaemia develops due to the inability of a narrowed coronary artery to meet an increased cardiac oxygen demand. Conversely, the **acute coronary syndromes (ACS)**, including in ascending order of severity, **unstable angina (UA)**, **non-ST segment elevation myocardial infarction (NSTEMI)** and **ST segment elevation myocardial infarction (STEMI)**, represent a spectrum of dangerous conditions in which myocardial ischaemia results from *a sudden decrease in the flow of blood through a coronary vessel*. This decrease is almost always initiated by the rupture of an atherosclerotic plaque, resulting in the formation of an intracoronary thrombus that diminishes or abolishes the flow of blood.

When a patient presents with suspected ACS, serial ECGs are immediately carried out. The hallmark of **STEMI** is *sustained elevation of the ST segments of the ECG* (Figure 42, upper left). This indicates that a large area of the myocardium, probably involving the full thickness of a ventricular wall, has developed a lesion as a result of prolonged ischaemia. Myocardial damage

releases intracellular proteins, such as **troponins T and I** into the blood. These serve as important markers of myocardial injury and as a prognostic tool. STEMI is confirmed when elevated levels of these markers are found in addition to the requisite ECG changes. STEMI typically occurs when a thrombus has completely occluded a coronary artery for a significant period of time, and usually causes more severe symptoms than do unstable angina or NSTEMI.

Incomplete or temporary coronary occlusion, or the existence of collateral coronary arteries that can maintain some supply of blood to the affected region, may result in a smaller degree of myocardial infarction (MI) and necrosis. This may not result in ST segment elevation, but does cause increased levels of cardiac markers of damage in the plasma. Patients with ACS who are found to have elevated levels of these markers, but who do not exhibit ST segment elevation, are deemed to have suffered an **NSTEMI**.

Patients who demonstrate symptoms associated with ACS, but who have neither ST segment elevation nor raised levels of troponins, are deemed to have **unstable angina**. In this case, it is likely

The Cardiovascular System at a Glance, Fourth Edition. Philip I. Aaronson, Jeremy P.T. Ward, and Michelle J. Connolly.

that the coronary obstruction has been of limited extent and/or duration (<20 min), and is thus sufficient to cause ischaemia but not detectable injury. Both NSTEMIs and UA may be associated with ECG changes other than ST elevation, for example ST segment depression and T-wave inversion.

Both NSTEMI and STEMI are grouped together as **acute MIs**, but are managed differently in the acute phase, in that reperfusion therapies, either pharmacological (thrombolysis), or preferably **percutaneous coronary intervention** is used to treat STEMI but not NSTEMI (see Chapters 43 and 45). Symptoms of UA/NSTEMI resemble those of stable angina, but they are frequently more painful, intense and persistent, often lasting at least 30 min. Pain is frequently unrelieved by glyceryl trinitrate. Typical presentations include:

1 Crescendo angina, where attacks are progressively more severe, prolonged and frequent
2 Angina of recent onset brought on by minimal exertion
3 Angina at rest/with minimal exertion or during sleep
4 Post-MI angina (ischaemic pain 24 h to 2 weeks after MI).

Pathophysiology of UA/NSTEMI

Studies have shown that episodes of unstable angina are preceded by a fall in coronary blood flow, thought to result from the periodic development of coronary **thrombosis** and **vasoconstriction**, which are triggered by coronary artery disease (Figure 42).

Thrombosis is promoted by the endothelial damage and turbulent blood flow associated with atherosclerotic plaques. Compared with the lesions of stable angina, plaques found in patients with ACS tend to have a thinner fibrous cap and a larger lipid core, and are generally more widespread and severe. These stenoses are often *eccentric* – the plaque does not surround the entire circumference of the artery. Such lesions are especially vulnerable to being ruptured by haemodynamic stress. This exposes the plaque interior, which powerfully stimulates platelet aggregation and thrombosis. The thrombus propagates out into the coronary lumen, occluding the artery. Rupture may also cause haemorrhage into the lesion itself, expanding it out into the lumen and worsening stenosis.

These events may be exacerbated by impaired coronary vasodilatation, and vasospasm due to plaque-associated endothelial damage, which reduces the local release of endothelium-dependent relaxing factors, such as nitric oxide. Platelet aggregation and thrombosis also cause the local generation of vasoconstrictors such as thromboxane A_2 and serotonin.

Risk stratification

The occurrence of UA and NSTEMI indicates that a patient has a high risk of undergoing subsequent episodes of coronary thrombosis which may cause more significant cardiac damage or death. In the USA, for example, ~4% of the 1.3 million people who enter hospital with UA/NSTEMI die within 30 days, and ~8% experience (re)infarction. Although NSTEMI is by definition a more serious 'event' than UA, in that myocardial necrosis has occurred, these are both heterogeneous conditions, and the risk of (re)infarction is higher in some patients with UA than in some with NSTEMI. Risk assessment is therefore of paramount importance.

Risk is scored on the basis of a number of factors, including frequency and severity of angina, elevated markers of cardiac necrosis, ECG changes (ST segment depression and/or T-wave inversion) and prior angiographic evidence of atherosclerotic plaque.

Management

UA/NSTEMI is a medical emergency. Patients are started on the 'ACS protocol', which consists of aggressive pharmacological therapy. This renders the acute coronary lesion less dangerous, minimizing residual ischaemia and reducing the likelihood of future coronary events. **Urgent revascularization** is considered for patients with high-risk and/or very significant coronary artery disease, or if drug treatment fails to control symptoms (see Chapter 43).

Drug treatment of UA/NSTEMI (see also Chapter 8 for drug mechanisms)

Antiplatelet therapy All patients with UA/NSTEMI are immediately treated with **300 mg aspirin**. This is then reduced to a smaller dose of 75 mg/day, which is continued for life. Aspirin is effective in treating ACS because it suppresses platelet aggregation, a key initial step in thrombosis. Clinical trials have shown that it reduces mortality or infarction by more than 50%.

The thienopyridine **clopidogrel**, which inhibits ADP-stimulated platelet aggregation, was shown in the 2000 CURE trial to reduce cardiovascular morbidity and mortality by ~20% in patients with UA/NSTEMI. Patients should be given 300 mg clopidogrel initially and then receive 75 mg/day for 12 months.

Antithrombin therapy Low molecular weight heparins (LMWHs) (e.g. dalteparin and similar drugs such as fondaparinux) which inhibit the coagulation cascade mainly at factor X and thrombin, are given to all patients with UA/NSTEMI. LMWH is given subcutaneously while patients are hospitalized, but not routinely thereafter.

Glycoprotein IIb/IIIa antagonists (e.g. tirofiban) are the most powerful of the antiplatelet drugs. These drugs are of proven benefit in UA/NSTEMI patients who receive percutaneous coronary intervention (PCI), a type of revascularization procedure in which plaque-stenosed coronary arteries are widened using a balloon catheter (see Chapter 43). PCI usually involves placing a medicated stent (a mesh tube) in the affected coronary to keep it open, and the glycoprotein IIb/IIIa antagonists reduce the tendency of stents to cause thrombosis.

Other drugs β-**Blockers** have been shown to reduce cardiovascular morbidity and mortality in patients with UA/NSTEMI, and should be given unless contraindicated (e.g. in moderate and severe asthma). **Nitrates** can be given, especially on a temporary basis, to relieve pain and to control symptoms of heart failure, but do not appear to reduce mortality. **Ca^{2+}-channel blockers** should *not* be used to treat UA/NSTEMI, although they may be continued if the patient is already receiving them for chronic stable angina. On the other hand, there is increasing evidence that **statins** and **angiotensin-converting enzyme inhibitors** improve survival in UA/NSTEMI.

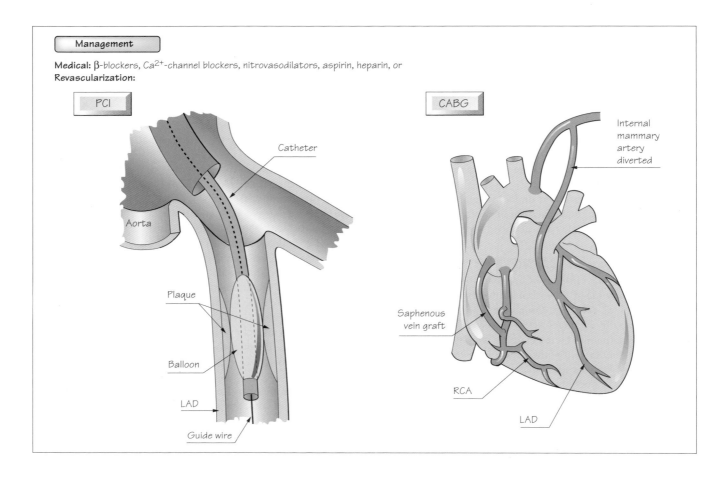

Management

Medical: β-blockers, Ca^{2+}-channel blockers, nitrovasodilators, aspirin, heparin, or
Revascularization:

PCI

Catheter

Aorta

Plaque

Balloon

LAD

Guide wire

CABG

Internal mammary artery diverted

Saphenous vein graft

RCA

LAD

Coronary artery bypass grafting (CABG) and **percutaneous coronary intervention (PCI)** are revascularization techniques that are used to treat patients with both stable angina and acute coronary syndromes. As described below, both procedures are used in higher risk patients, with the choice of technique determined by several factors including severity of disease and the wishes of the individual. It is estimated that in 2003 CABG and PCI were carried out on approximately 270 000 and 650 000 patients in the USA, respectively.

CABG is a surgical procedure (Figure 43, right) which was introduced in the 1960s. Initially, CABG mainly involved the use of lengths of healthy superfluous blood vessels (conduits) which were removed and then attached (anastamosed) between the aorta and the coronary arteries distal to the stenosis, thus allowing a supply of blood to the heart that bypassed the obstruction. Conduits commonly used for CABG included **saphenous vein** segments harvested from the leg. However, these have limited long-term patency due to early postoperative thrombosis, intimal hyperpla-

sia with smooth muscle proliferation within the first year, and the development of atherosclerosis after approximately 5–7 years. For this reason, the **left internal thoracic (**also termed **mammary) artery** (LITA) is now used for grafting much more widely than the saphenous vein. In general, the LITA is not disconnected from its parent (subclavian) artery, but is cut distally and attached to the coronary artery. Unlike the saphenous vein, 90–95% of LITA grafts remain patent after 10 years, and patients with a LITA graft to the crucial left anterior descending coronary artery have improved long-term survival compared with patients receiving saphenous vein grafts. If multivessel disease is present, the use of LITA and saphenous vein grafts can be combined. More recently, the use of both left and right internal thoracic arteries (**bilateral internal thoracic artery**) for grafting has become more common, especially for younger patients. For example, the right internal thoracic artery may be grafted to the left anterior descending coronary artery while the LITA is anastomosed to the circumflex system. The gastroepiploic and radial arteries can also be used for grafting.

The Cardiovascular System at a Glance, Fourth Edition. Philip I. Aaronson, Jeremy P.T. Ward, and Michelle J. Connolly.

CABG is usually perform with the patient on *cardiopulmonary bypass*, with the heart stopped. Blood is typically removed from the right atrium, drained into a reservoir, and then pumped through an oxygenator, then a filter and back into the aorta to perfuse the systemic circulation. The main complications of the procedure are a systemic inflammatory response, atrial fibrillation and persistent neurological abnormalities. These latter are thought to be caused by emboli, either formed in the bypass circuit or produced by disturbance of aortic plaques during cannulation, which lodge in the cerebral vasculature. These complications can be avoided by *off-pump CABG*, which does not involve stopping the heart. In this case, the region of the cardiac wall encompassing the target coronary segment is immobilized to allow grafting. Randomized trials show that both types of CABG offer similar outcomes. The mortality rate associated with CABG is ~2%.

PCI, first used in 1977, is a much less invasive procedure. A guiding catheter is introduced via the femoral, brachial or radial artery, and is positioned near the target stenosis. A guiding wire is then advanced down the lumen of the coronary artery until it is positioned across the stenosis. A balloon catheter is advanced over this wire, and then inflated at the site of the stenosis to increase the luminal diameter (Figure 43, left). Emergency CABG is required in 1–2% of patients due to acute vessel closure after this procedure. PCI is judged a success if the arterial lumen at the stenosis is increased to more than 50% of the normal coronary artery diameter.

Restenosis at the site of the PCI occurs within 6 months of the procedure in 30% of patients. Restenosis can be caused by elastic recoil of the vessel or by **intimal hyperplasia**, a thickening of the inner layer of the artery which is initiated by endothelial denudation, and which involves proliferation of intimal smooth muscle cells and the production of connective tissue. Restenosis generally causes a return of cardiac ischaemia and angina, in which case PCI is repeated or CABG is performed.

Stents were first introduced in 1986 in an attempt to prevent elastic recoil and restenosis. Stents are cylindrical metal (e.g. stainless steel, platinum) mesh or slotted tubes that are implanted into the artery at the site of balloon expansion following angioplasty. They are mainly used in vessels >3 mm in diameter and are designed either to be self-expanding, or to be expanded by the catheter balloon, so that they press out against the inner wall of the coronary artery, holding it open. Stenting is currently being used in ~90% of PCI procedures as its introduction has substantially improved acute PCI success, has reduced the rate of restenosis to ~15%, and has correspondingly decreased the need for repeat revascularizations. Various approaches are being tried to reduce this 'in-stent' restenosis still further. Notably, the 2002 RAVEL trial assessed the use of stents that were coated with the proliferation-inhibiting drug **rapamycin** (sirolimus), which gradually eluted from the stent over a month. Rapamycin caused a dramatic decrease in restenosis, and virtually abolished the need for another revascularization over the year following the procedure. Subsequent studies have shown that the use of drug-eluting stents reduces the incidence of major adverse cardiac events during the 9 months following PCI by ~50%, so that drug-eluting stents utiliz-ing rapamycin as well as the alternative agents **paclitaxel** and **everolimus** are now used routinely.

The main potential complication arising from stenting is thrombosis, which can be well controlled with aspirin and clopidogrel. Routine PCI bears a risk of mortality of ≤1%.

Revascularization vs medical management: which patients benefit?

In general, revascularization is preferred for patients who are at high risk of developing worsening ischaemic heart disease and/or acute coronary syndromes, or in whom pharmacological treatment is either not controlling ischaemic symptoms (e.g. angina) or is causing intolerable side effects. Particularly important indications for revascularization in *stable angina* include the presence of significant plaques in three coronary arteries (particularly when the left anterior descending, which perfuses the largest fraction of the myocardium, is involved) and reduced left ventricular function, which indicates the presence of chronic ongoing ischaemia.

Revascularization is also very frequently used in *UA/NSTEMI* (see Chapter 42), and is recommended for patients who are judged to be at moderate or high risk for death or myocardial infarction, as judged by various indices relating to the seriousness of their signs and symptoms. Revascularization is now also preferred over thrombolysis to produce immediate coronary reperfusion during acute myocardial infarction (STEMI; see Chapters 43 and 45). In *heart failure*, revascularization can be used to reperfuse a region of 'hibernating myocardium', in which cells are still alive but are contracting poorly because they are chronically ischaemic.

PCI vs CABG

PCI is preferred when one or two arteries are diseased, as long as the disease is not too diffuse and the plaques are amenable to this approach. CABG is used when all three main coronary arteries are diseased (triple vessel disease), when the left coronary mainstem has a significant stenosis, when the lesion is not amenable to PCI, and when left ventricular function is poor. CABG has been shown to reduce angina symptoms more than does PCI in the first 5 years after the procedure, but symptoms tend to return gradually over the years in either case, and eventually recur similarly after both procedures. Revascularization must be repeated much more often after PCI than CABG, although improvements in stenting will probably narrow this difference. The use of PCI is growing rapidly, while that of CABG is diminishing.

Benefits of revascularization

Compared with medical therapy, CABG improves survival in patients with severe atherosclerotic disease in all three major coronary arteries or a more than 50% stenosis of the left main coronary artery, particularly if left ventricular function is impaired. Compared with medical therapy, PCI does not improve survival. However, PCI results in a greater improvement of angina symptoms and exercise tolerance than does medical therapy, and also diminishes the need for drugs.

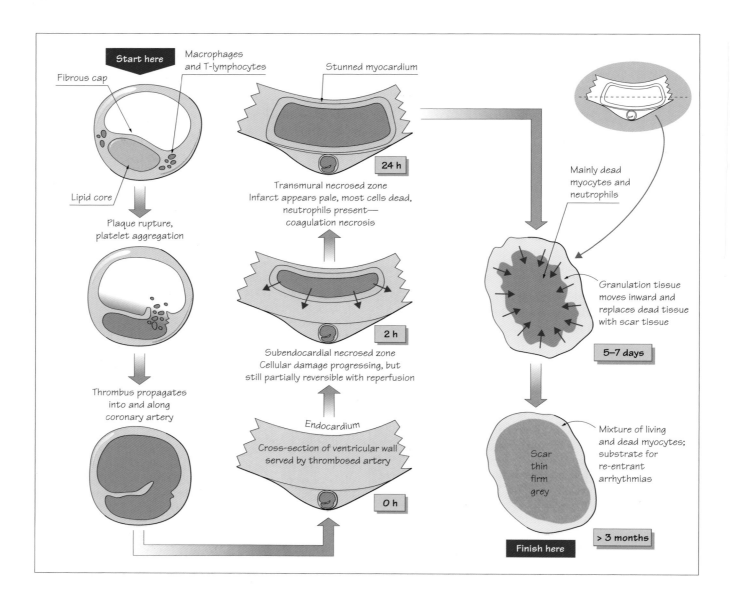

Infarction is tissue death caused by ischaemia. Acute **myocardial infarction** (MI) occurs when localized myocardial ischaemia causes the development of a defined region of **necrosis**. MI is most often caused by rupture of an atherosclerotic lesion in a coronary artery. This causes the formation of a thrombus that plugs the artery, stopping it from supplying blood to the region of the heart that it supplies.

Role of thrombosis in MI

Pivotal studies by DeWood and colleagues showed that *coronary thrombosis* is the critical event resulting in MI. Of patients presenting within 4 h of symptom onset with ECG evidence of transmural MI, coronary angiography showed that 87% had complete thrombotic occlusion of the infarct-related artery. The incidence of total occlusion fell to 65% 12–24 h after symptom onset due to sponta-

neous fibrinolysis. Fresh thrombi on top of ruptured plaques have also been demonstrated in the infarct-related arteries in patients dying of MI.

Mechanisms and consequences of plaque rupture

Coronary plaques that are prone to rupture are typically small and non-obstructive, with a large lipid-rich core covered by a thin fibrous cap. These 'high-risk' plaques typically contain abundant **macrophages** and **T lymphocytes** which are thought to release **metalloproteases** and **cytokines** that weaken the fibrous cap, rendering it liable to tear or erode due to the shear stress exerted by the blood flow.

Plaque rupture reveals subendothelial collagen, which serves as a site of platelet adhesion, activation and aggregation. This results in:

The Cardiovascular System at a Glance, Fourth Edition. Philip I. Aaronson, Jeremy P.T. Ward, and Michelle J. Connolly.

1 The release of substances such as *thromboxane A₂ (TXA₂)*, *fibrinogen, 5-hydroxytryptamine (5-HT), platelet activating factor* and *adenosine diphosphate (ADP)*, which further promote platelet aggregation.

2 Activation of the clotting cascade, leading to fibrin formation and propagation and stabilization of the occlusive thrombus.

The endothelium is often damaged around areas of coronary artery disease. The resulting deficit of antithrombotic factors such as *thrombomodulin* and *prostacyclin* enhances thrombus formation. In addition, the tendency of several platelet-derived factors (e.g. TXA₂, 5-HT) to cause vasoconstriction is increased in the absence of endothelial-derived relaxing factors. This may promote the development of local vasospasm, which worsens coronary occlusion.

Sudden death and acute coronary syndrome onset show a **circadian variation** (daily cycle), peaking at around 9 a.m. with a trough at around 11 p.m. Levels of catecholamines peak about an hour after awakening in the morning, resulting in maximal levels of platelet aggregability, vascular tone, heart rate and blood pressure, which may trigger plaque rupture and thrombosis. Increased physical and mental stress can also cause MI and sudden death, supporting a role for increases in catecholamines in MI pathophysiology. Furthermore, chronic β-adrenergic receptor blockade abolishes the circadian rhythm of MI.

Autopsies of young subjects killed in road accidents often show small plaque ruptures in susceptible arteries, suggesting that plaque rupture does not always have pathological consequences. The degree of coronary occlusion and myocardial damage caused by plaque rupture probably depends on systemic catecholamine levels, as well as local factors such as plaque location and morphology, the depth of plaque rupture and the extent to which coronary vasoconstriction occurs.

Severe and prolonged ischaemia produces a region of necrosis spanning the entire thickness of the myocardial wall. Such a *transmural* infarct usually causes ST segment elevation (i.e. STEMI; see Chapter 45). Less severe and protracted ischaemia can arise when:

1 Coronary occlusion is followed by spontaneous reperfusion

2 The infarct-related artery is not completely occluded

3 Occlusion is complete, but an existing collateral blood supply prevents complete ischaemia

4 The oxygen demand in the affected zone of myocardium is smaller.

Under these conditions, the necrotic zone may be mainly limited to the subendocardium, typically causing non-ST segment elevation MI.

The classification of acute MI according to the presence or absence of ST segment elevation is designed to allow rapid decision-making concerning whether thrombolysis should be initiated (see Chapter 43). This classification replaces the previous one, based on the presence or absence of Q waves on the ECG, which was less useful for guiding immediate therapy.

Evolution of the infarct

Both infarcted and unaffected myocardial regions undergo progressive changes over the hours, days and weeks following coronary thrombosis. This process of postinfarct myocardial evolution leads to the occurrence of characteristic complications at predictable times after the initial event (see Chapter 45).

Ischaemia causes an immediate loss of contractility in the affected myocardium, a condition termed **hypokinesis**. Necrosis starts to develop in the subendocardium (which is most prone to ischaemia; see Chapter 2), about 15–30 min after coronary occlusion. The necrotic region grows outward towards the epicardium over the next 3–6 h, eventually spanning the entire ventricular wall. In some areas (generally at the edges of the infarct) the myocardium is **stunned** (reversibly damaged) but will eventually recover if blood flow is restored. Contractility in the remaining viable myocardium increases, a process termed **hyperkinesis**.

A progression of cellular, histological and gross changes develop within the infarct. Although alterations in the gross appearance of infarcted tissue are not apparent for at least 6 h after the onset of cell death, cell biochemistry and ultrastructure begin to show abnormalities within 20 min. Cell damage is progressive, becomingly increasingly irreversible over about 12 h. This period therefore provides a window of opportunity during which percutaneous coronary intervention (PCI) or thrombolysis leading to reperfusion may salvage some of the infarct (see Chapter 43).

Between 4 and 12 h after cell death starts, the infarcted myocardium begins to undergo **coagulation necrosis**, a process characterized by cell swelling, organelle breakdown and protein denaturation. After about 18 h, **neutrophils** (phagocytic lymphocytes) enter the infarct. Their numbers reach a peak after about 5 days, and then decline. After 3–4 days, **granulation tissue** appears at the edges of the infarct zone. This consists of **macrophages**, **fibroblasts**, which lay down scar tissue, and **new capillaries**. The infarcted myocardium is especially soft between 4 and 7 days, and is therefore maximally prone to **rupturing**. This event is usually fatal, may occur at any time during the first 2 weeks, and is responsible for about 10% of MI mortality. As the granulation tissue migrates inward toward the centre of the infarct over several weeks, the necrotic tissue is engulfed and digested by the macrophages. The granulation tissue then progressively matures, with an increase in connective (scar) tissue and loss of capillaries. After 2–3 months, the infarct has healed, leaving a non-contracting region of the ventricular wall that is thinned, firm and pale grey.

Infarct expansion, the stretching and thinning of the infarcted wall, may occur within the first day or so after an MI, especially if the infarction is large or transmural, or has an anterior location. Over the course of several months, there is progressive dilatation, not only of the infarct zone, but also of healthy myocardium. This process of **ventricular remodelling** is caused by an increase in end-diastolic wall stress. Infarct expansion puts patients at a substantial risk for the development of congestive heart failure, ventricular arrhythmias and free wall rupture.

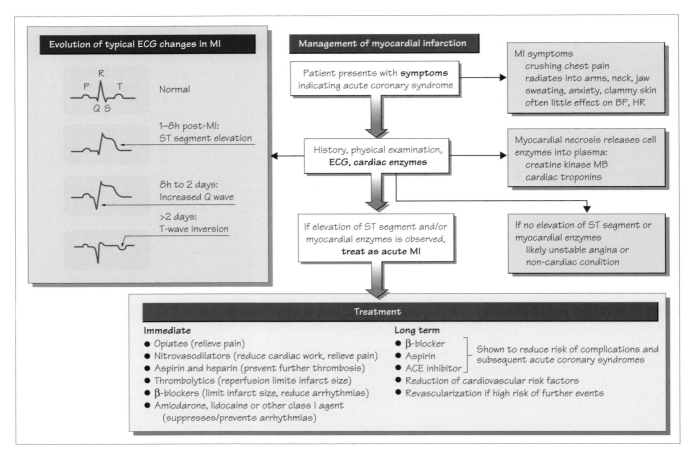

Evolution of typical ECG changes in MI

Normal

1–8h post-MI:
ST segment elevation

8h to 2 days:
Increased Q wave

>2 days:
T-wave inversion

Management of myocardial infarction

Patient presents with **symptoms** indicating acute coronary syndrome

MI symptoms
  crushing chest pain
  radiates into arms, neck, jaw
  sweating, anxiety, clammy skin
  often little effect on BP, HR

History, physical examination, **ECG, cardiac enzymes**

Myocardial necrosis releases cell enzymes into plasma:
  creatine kinase MB
  cardiac troponins

If elevation of ST segment and/or myocardial enzymes is observed, **treat as acute MI**

If no elevation of ST segment or myocardial enzymes
  likely unstable angina or
  non-cardiac condition

Treatment

Immediate
- Opiates (relieve pain)
- Nitrovasodilators (reduce cardiac work, relieve pain)
- Aspirin and heparin (prevent further thrombosis)
- Thrombolytics (reperfusion limits infarct size)
- β-blockers (limit infarct size, reduce arrhythmias)
- Amiodarone, lidocaine or other class I agent (suppresses/prevents arrhythmias)

Long term
- β-blocker
- Aspirin   Shown to reduce risk of complications and subsequent acute coronary syndromes
- ACE inhibitor
- Reduction of cardiovascular risk factors
- Revascularization if high risk of further events

Symptoms and signs

Patients usually present with sudden onset central crushing chest pain, which may radiate down either arm (but more commonly the left) to the jaw, back or neck. The pain lasts longer than 20 min and is not relieved by glyceryl trinitrate (GTN). The pain is often associated with dyspnoea, nausea, sweatiness and palpitations. Intense feelings of impending doom (*angor animi*) are common. Some individuals present atypically, with no symptoms (**silent infarct**, most common in diabetic patients with diabetic neuropathy), unusual locations of the pain, syncope or pulmonary oedema. The pulse may demonstrate a tachycardia or bradycardia. The blood pressure is usually normal. The rest of the cardiovascular system examination may be unremarkable, but there may be a third or fourth heart sound audible on auscultation as well as a new and/or worsening murmur, which may be due to papillary muscle rupture in the left heart.

Investigations

- **ECG:** ECG changes associated with myocardial infarction (MI) indicate the site and thickness of the infarct. The first ECG change is peaking of the T wave. ST segment elevation then follows rapidly in a ST elevation myocardial infarction (STEMI).
- **Troponin I:** elevated plasma concentrations of troponin I indicates that myocardial necrosis has occurred. Troponins begin to

rise within 3–12 h of the onset of chest pain and peak at 24–48 h and then clear in about 2 weeks. It is important that a troponin level is interpreted in the clinical context, because conditions other than MI can damage cardiac muscle (e.g. heart failure, myocarditis, pericarditis, pulmonary embolism or renal failure). Patients presenting with suspected acute coronary syndromes (ACS) should have troponin measured at presentation. If it is negative, it should be repeated 12 hours later. If the 12 h troponin is also negative, then MI but not unstable angina can be excluded.

Management

Immediate In the ambulance or on first medical contact, individuals with suspected MI are immediately given 300 mg chewable **aspirin** and 300 mg **clopidogrel** to block further platelet aggregation. Two puffs of **GTN** are sprayed underneath the tongue. The patient is assessed by brief history and a clinical examination, and a 12-lead ECG is recorded. The patient is given oxygen via a face mask. **Morphine**, which has vasodilator properties, together with an anti-emetic (e.g. metoclopramide) is administered to relieve pain and anxiety, thus reducing the tachycardia that these cause. A **β-blocker** (e.g. metoprolol) should be given unless contraindicated (e.g. LV failure or moderate to severe asthma) because β-blockers decrease infarct size and have a positive effect on mortality. The preferred treatment of a confirmed STEMI is revascularization with **percutaneous coronary intervention** (see Chapter 43) of the blocked artery within 2h of symptom onset. Ideally, every hospital would be equipped with the ability to perform percutaneous coronary intervention (PCI) but in reality this is not the case. However, those that do not have the capacity for PCI are affiliated with centres that do and protocols exist to enable the rapid transfer of patients. If it is not possible to get the patient to a centre for PCI in less than 2h from symptom onset, the alternative is pharmacological dissolution of the clot with thrombolytic agents within 12h of presentation unless contraindicated (see below). There are specific ECG criteria for the diagnosis of STEMI and use of thrombolysis: *ST segment elevation* of >1mm in two or more limb leads or >2mm in two or more chest leads, or *new onset left bundle branch block*, or *posterior changes* (ST depression and tall R waves in leads V1–V3). If thrombolysis fails, the patient must be sent for rescue PCI to be performed as soon as possible.

Subsequent Long-term treatment with aspirin, a β-blocker and an angiotensin-converting enzyme inhibitor (**ACEI**) reduces the complications of MI and the risk of reinfarction. Cessation of smoking, control of hypertension and diabetes, and reduction of lipids using a **statin** (see Chapter 36) are vital.

Thrombolytic agents

Thrombolysis is the dissolution of the blood clot plugging the infarct-related coronary artery. As described in Chapter 43, thrombolytic agents induce **fibrinolysis**, the fragmentation of the fibrin strands holding the clot together. This permits *reperfusion* of the ischaemic zone. Reperfusion limits infarct size and reduces the risk of complications such as infarct expansion, arrhythmias and cardiac failure. Clinical trials, notably ISIS-2 (1988), have demonstrated that thrombolytic agents reduce mortality by about 25% in STEMI, although patients without ST elevation (i.e. NSTEMI) do *not* benefit from thrombolysis. It is critical that thrombolysis is instituted as quickly as possible. Although significant reductions in mortality occur when thrombolytics are given within 12h of symptom onset, the greatest benefits occur when therapy is instituted within 2h ('time is muscle').

The two main agents for thrombolysis are **streptokinase (SK)** and **tissue plasminogen activator (tPA)** (see Chapter 43). tPA appears to have a slight survival benefit over SK, but the former is much less expensive. tPA is very quickly cleared from the plasma, and **reteplase** and **tenecteplase** are newer agents that have been made by modifying the structure of tPA in order to impede plasma clearance. Both can therefore be given by bolus injection by paramedics, thus facilitating prehospital thrombolysis.

The main risk of thrombolysis is bleeding, particularly intracerebral haemorrhage, which occurs in ~1% of cases. Contraindications to thrombolysis therefore include recent haemorrhagic stroke, recent surgery or trauma, and severe hypertension.

Other drugs used in acute myocardial infarction

Antiplatelet and **anticoagulant** therapy is used after MI to prevent further platelet aggregation and thrombosis. The ISIS-2 trial demonstrated a 23% reduction in 35-day mortality in patients randomized to aspirin. Combined aspirin and SK had an additive benefit compared with placebo (42% reduction). Following an initial 300mg loading dose, 75mg/day aspirin should be given thereafter for life to all patients to prevent vessel occlusion and infarction. Because tPA, reteplase and tenecteplase are more fibrin-specific than SK, intravenous heparin should be given for a duration of 48–72h to reduce the risk of further thrombosis when these agents are administered, or when the patient is at high risk of developing systemic emboli (e.g. with anterior MI or atrial fibrillation).

β-Blockers are beneficial in MI for several reasons. They diminish O_2 demand by lowering heart rate and decrease ventricular wall stress by lowering afterload. They therefore reduce ischaemia and infarct size when given acutely. They also decrease recurrent ischaemia and free wall rupture, and suppress arrhythmias (see Chapter 48). Long-term oral β-blockade reduces mortality, recurrent MI and sudden death by about 25%.

ACEI (e.g. lisinopril, ramipril) reduce afterload and ventricular wall stress and improve ejection fraction. Inhibition of ACE raises bradykinin levels, which may improve endothelial function and limit coronary vasospasm. ACEI also limit ventricular remodelling and infarct expansion (see Chapter 47), thereby reducing mortality and the incidence of congestive heart failure and recurrent MI. Therapy should be instituted within 24h in patients with STEMI, especially if there is evidence of heart failure or left ventricular dysfunction, and should continue long term if LV dysfunction remains evident.

Complications of acute myocardial infarction

There are two main groups of complications associated with acute MI: mechanical and arrhythmic.

With large infarcts (>20–25% of the left ventricle) depression of pump function is sufficient to cause **cardiac failure**. An infarct involving more than 40% of the LV causes cardiogenic shock. **Rupture** of the free LV wall is almost always fatal. Severe LV failure (cardiogenic shock) as a result of MI is heralded by a large fall in cardiac output, pulmonary congestion and often hypotension. The mortality is extremely high. Treatment involves O_2 to prevent hypoxaemia, diamorphine for pain and anxiety, fluid resuscitation to optimize filling pressure and positive inotropes (e.g. the β_1-agonist dobutamine) are infused to aid myocardial contractility. Revascularization is crucial. **Intraortic balloon counterpulsation** can be used temporarily to support the circulation. A catheter-mounted balloon is inserted via the femoral artery and positioned in the descending thoracic aorta. The balloon is inflated during diastole, increasing the pressure in the aortic arch and thereby improving perfusion of the coronary and cerebral arteries. During systole, deflation of the balloon creates a suction effect that reduces ventricular afterload and promotes systemic perfusion.

Rupture of the ventricular septum creates a **ventricular septal defect** (VSD) and may result in leakage of blood between the ventricles. Rupture of the myocardium underlying a papillary muscle, or more rarely of the papillary muscle itself, may cause **mitral regurgitation**, detected clinically as a pansystolic murmur radiating to the axilla. **Dressler's syndrome** is the triad of pericarditis, pericardial effusion and fever.

Arrhythmias in the acute phase include ventricular ectopic beats, and the potentially life-threatening broad complex (QRS complex >0.12s) tachyarrhythmias, ventricular tachycardia (VT) or ventricular fibrillation (VF). Supraventricular arrhythmias include atrial ectopics, atrial flutter and atrial fibrillation. Bradyarrhythmias are also common, including sinus bradycardia, and first-, second- and third-degree AV block. **Infarct expansion** (see Chapter 44) is a dangerous late complication.

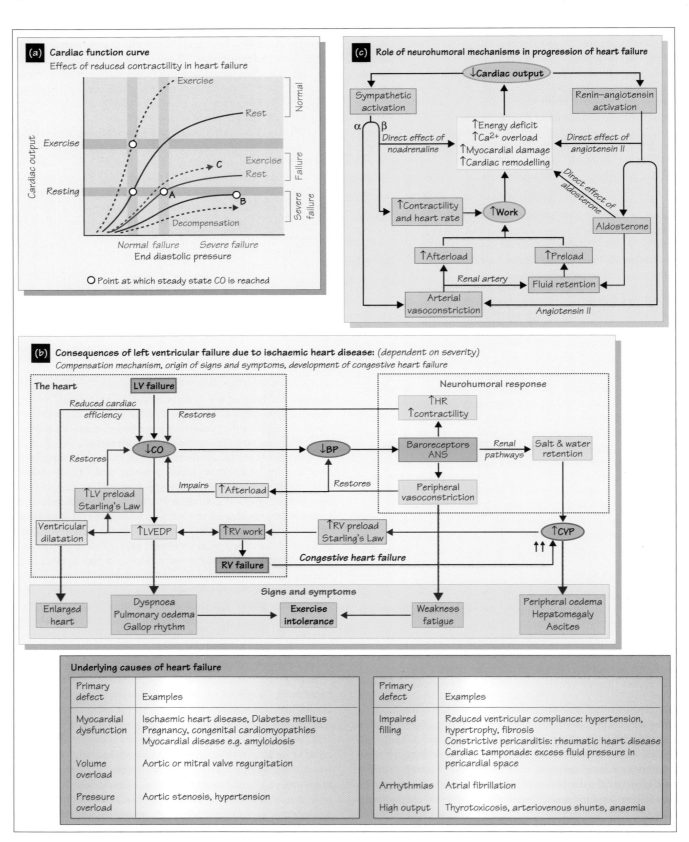

(a) Cardiac function curve
Effect of reduced contractility in heart failure

O Point at which steady state CO is reached

(c) Role of neurohumoral mechanisms in progression of heart failure

(b) Consequences of left ventricular failure due to ischaemic heart disease: (dependent on severity)
Compensation mechanism, origin of signs and symptoms, development of congestive heart failure

Underlying causes of heart failure

Primary defect	Examples		Primary defect	Examples
Myocardial dysfunction	Ischaemic heart disease, Diabetes mellitus Pregnancy, congenital cardiomyopathies Myocardial disease e.g. amyloidosis		Impaired filling	Reduced ventricular compliance: hypertension, hypertrophy, fibrosis Constrictive pericarditis: rheumatic heart disease Cardiac tamponade: excess fluid pressure in pericardial space
Volume overload	Aortic or mitral valve regurgitation		Arrhythmias	Atrial fibrillation
Pressure overload	Aortic stenosis, hypertension		High output	Thyrotoxicosis, arteriovenous shunts, anaemia

The Cardiovascular System at a Glance, Fourth Edition. Philip I. Aaronson, Jeremy P.T. Ward, and Michelle J. Connolly.

Chronic heart failure is a complex and progressive disorder that occurs when the heart is incapable of generating sufficient cardiac output (CO) to meet the demands of the body. Initially, compensatory mechanisms may allow adequate CO to be maintained at rest but not during exercise (**exercise intolerance**). Eventually CO cannot be maintained at rest (**decompensation**); this can be precipitated by acute illness (e.g. influenza), stress or drugs (e.g. NSAIDs). Chronic heart failure is predominantly a disease of old age. It occurs in ~2% of patients under 50 years, but >10% over 65; 5-year survival is <50%. **Acute heart failure** describes a sudden loss of cardiac function, for example **acute coronary syndrome** (see Chapter 44). It may cause pulmonary congestion and oedema (see below) and cardiogenic shock (see Chapter 31).

Causes of heart failure

The most common cause (~70% cases) is impaired ventricular contraction with an **ejection fraction** <45% (**systolic failure**; Figure 46a), generally a consequence of ischaemic heart disease (IHD). **Diastolic failure** is due to impaired filling, caused by reduced ventricular **compliance** (*flexibility*; e.g. fibrosis, hypertrophy), restriction (e.g. pericarditis) or impaired relaxation (see below). Ejection fraction may be normal or increased. Systolic failure is generally accompanied by diastolic failure, while the latter can occur alone. Both involve increased filling pressures, so have similar clinical manifestations.

As IHD generally affects the left ventricle, **left heart failure** is most common, and is associated with **dyspnoea** (breathlessness), an **enlarged heart** and **fatigue** (see below). **Right heart failure** may result from chronic lung disease (**cor pulmonale**), pulmonary hypertension or embolism, and valve disease, but usually it is secondary to left heart failure (**congestive** or *biventricular* **heart failure**) (Figure 46b). Central venous pressure (CVP) is greatly increased, with consequent jugular venous distension, swelling of the liver (**hepatomegaly**), **peripheral oedema** and peritoneal fluid accumulation (**ascites**).

High output failure occurs when a healthy heart is unable to meet grossly elevated demands for output due to anaemia or a drastically reduced peripheral resistance (e.g. septic shock).

Pathophysiology

The pathophysiology of chronic heart failure is largely a consequence of mechanisms that compensate for reduced cardiac function. Impaired cardiac function causes accumulation of venous blood and thus raised filling pressures, so CO increases as a consequence of **Starling's law** (Figure 46a,b; see Chapter 17). **Neurohumoral** mechanisms are activated by the **baroreceptor reflex** (Figure 46c; see Chapter 28), and the autonomic nervous system and circulating catecholamines stimulate increases in heart rate and contractility, arterial vasoconstriction (raises TPR) and venoconstriction (raises CVP) (see Chapters 12 and 17). Sympathetic stimulation of renal granular cells and reduced renal perfusion cause release of **renin**, and consequently **angiotensin II** and **aldosterone; vasopressin** (antidiuretic hormone, ADH) also increases. These cause renal sodium and water retention and so elevate blood volume and CVP (and thus CO through Starling's law) (see Chapter 29). Angiotensin II and vasopressin also increase TPR. In mild disease these mechanisms can maintain CO and blood pressure without overt symptoms. However, end-diastolic pressure (EDP) and volume (EDV) are always elevated (Figure 46a, A) so **ejection fraction** is reduced, an early sign of heart failure.

As cardiac function declines, CO can only be maintained by an ever-increasing CVP and heart rate (Figure 46a, B), fostering further **myocardial damage** (see below). This vicious circle drives a relentless decay towards decompensation and death. Although adequate CO may be maintained at rest even in quite severe failure, this is at the expense of greatly increased venous pressures as the function curve flattens and Starling's law becomes less effective (Figure 46a, A,B; see Chapter 17). High venous pressures underlie most signs and symptoms of heart failure.

Consequences of compensation (Figure 46b)

Initially, symptoms only appear during exertion, which exacerbates the rise in venous pressures (Figure 46a, C); this limits the ability to exercise (**exercise intolerance**). Any increase in contractility and heart rate during exercise is small because they are already strongly stimulated at rest, and in late disease β-adrenoceptor density and sensitivity are reduced. **Dyspnoea** on exertion is often the first symptom of left heart failure. It is caused by **pulmonary congestion** due to the raised pulmonary venous pressure, making the lungs stiffer and so promoting the sensation of breathlessness. Redistribution of blood to the lungs on lying down or during sleep can instigate dyspnoea (**orthopnoea; paroxysmal nocturnal dyspnoea**), and in severe failure and decompensation **pulmonary oedema**, when fluid enters the alveoli. This is a life-threatening condition causing extreme dyspnoea and hypoxaemia.

A high CVP similarly causes **peripheral oedema** (see Chapter 21), **hepatomegaly** and **ascites**, common features of **right** and **congestive heart failure**. High EDP eventually lead to **cardiac dilation** and a greatly enlarged heart (see below), and is associated with an **S₃/S₄** gallop rhythm (see Chapter 16). In more severe disease diversion of blood flow from skeletal muscle and non-essential tissues leads to **weakness** and **fatigue**, and contributes to exercise intolerance.

Myocardial dysfunction and remodelling

Chronic heart failure is characterized by progressive cardiac dysfunction, accompanied by **myocardial remodelling**.

Compensation forces an already compromised heart to work harder. This leads to **energy deficit**, dysfunction of ATP-dependent transporters (e.g. Ca^{2+}-ATPases and Na^+ pump) (see Chapters 10 and 12), and consequent **Ca^{2+} overload** (Figure 46c). This impairs relaxation and fosters lengthening of the action potential (e.g. *acquired long QT syndrome*; see Chapter 54) and generation of **arrhythmias**, a major cause of sudden death. Mitochondrial dysfunction worsens the energy deficit. **Oxidative stress**, and cytokines promote further damage, structural alterations and **apoptosis** (programmed cell death). Myocardial remodelling is potentiated by direct action of noradrenaline, angiotensin II and aldosterone (Figure 46c).

Dilatation reduces cardiac *efficiency*, as pressure in a sphere is proportional to wall tension (i.e. myocardial force) divided by radius (Law of Laplace). Large dilated hearts therefore have to contract harder in order to develop the same pressure as smaller hearts.

Cardiac dilatation must not be confused with **hypertrophy**, where cardiac myocytes grow larger and ventricular wall thickness increases in response to a sustained increase in afterload (e.g. hypertension, aortic stenosis). Hypertrophy is not usually associated with IHD. Although force is increased, the thicker ventricle is less **compliant**, which impedes filling and contributes to *diastolic failure*. **Capillary density** is reduced, lowering **coronary reserve** (difference between maximum and resting coronary flow), so myocardial perfusion may be limited. Changes in **contractile protein isoforms** (myosin, tropomyosin) decrease contraction velocity and contractility. Gross hypertrophy may physically impair valve operation.

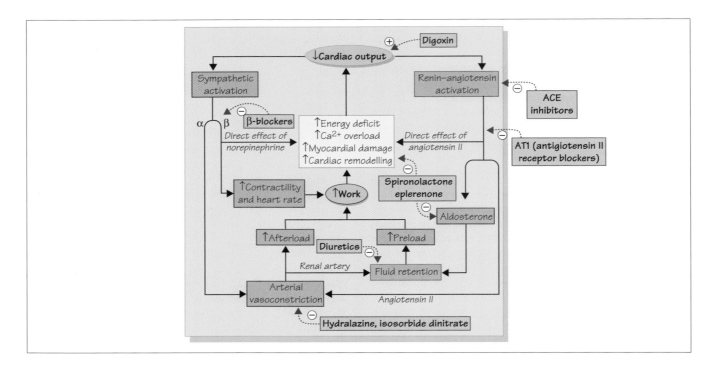

Therapy of chronic heart failure (CHF) is designed to: (i) improve the quality of life by reducing symptoms; (ii) lengthen survival; and (iii) slow the progression of cardiac deterioration. CHF typically has an underlying cause such as ischaemic heart disease, and may be exacerbated by specific **precipitating factors** such as infection or arrhythmias, as well as by myocardial abnormalities which develop as CHF progresses (e.g. valvular dysfunction). As well as the symptoms of CHF per se, both underlying and precipitating factors should, if possible, be treated. Restricting activity and reducing dietary sodium help to lessen cardiac workload and fluid retention.

The **sympathetic** and **renin–angiotensin–aldosterone** (RAA) systems activated in response to reduced pump function initially help to maintain cardiac output, but also drive the progression of cardiac deterioration (Figure 47; see also Chapter 46). Therapy mainly involves inhibiting these systems, and is initiated with **angiotensin-converting enzyme inhibitors (ACEI)** or **β-blockers**, which slow CHF progression, lengthen survival time and improve haemodynamic parameters. **Angiotensin receptor blockers (ARBs)** are used as an alternative in patients who cannot tolerate ACEI. If symptoms are not adequately controlled with one of these three types of drugs, one of the other classes is then also prescribed. Typically, a drug targeting the RAA system is combined with a β-blocker, although the ACEI–ARB combination can be used in β-blocker intolerant patients. Combining all three classes has been shown not to be beneficial and potentially increases side effects, so is not recommended. A **diuretic** can also be used to control fluid accumulation and **digoxin** may be used to support cardiac function and reduce symptoms. In severe or refractory CHF, or when existing therapy fails to control symptoms adequately, an **aldosterone antagonist** such as spironolactone or eplerenone is recommended.

Positive inotropes such as **dobutamine**, **dopamine** or **milrinone** may be used temporarily if decompensation (an acute worsening of heart failure) occurs, as can **intra-aortic balloon counterpulsation** (see Chapter 45).

Device therapy is playing an increasingly important role in treating chronic heart failure. **Implantable cardiac defibrillators** are used in many patients with moderate to severe CHF, as ~50% of patients will have sudden cardiac death, which is mainly caused by ventricular fibrillation (see Chapter 50). **Cardiac resynchronization therapy,** which involves implantation of a pacemaker that stimulates both ventricles to contract simultaneously, can also be used in patients with moderate to severe CHF who show evidence of asynchronous ventricular contraction.

A **ventricular assist device** (a pump that takes over part or all of the heart's pumping action) can be used as a bridge for patients awaiting cardiac transplant, or as a destination device to lengthen survival if transplant is not possible.

ACEI and other vasodilators

As described in Chapter 29, angiotension II causes vasoconstriction and promotes fluid retention via multiple mechanisms. ACEI, which inhibit the conversion of angiotensin I to angiotensin II, therefore dilate arteries and veins, and reduce blood volume and oedema. Arterial vasodilatation decreases afterload and cardiac work, and improves tissue perfusion by increasing stroke volume and cardiac output. Venous dilatation and reduction of fluid retention diminish pulmonary congestion, oedema and central venous pressure (CVP) (preload). Reduction of preload lowers ventricular filling pressure, therefore lowering cardiac wall stress, workload and ischaemia. ACEI also delay abnormal cardiac hypertrophy and fibrosis, which are thought to be promoted by angiotensin II.

The Cardiovascular System at a Glance, Fourth Edition. Philip I. Aaronson, Jeremy P.T. Ward, and Michelle J. Connolly.

Angiotensin (AT1) receptor blockers such as **losartan** are used in patients unable to tolerate the cough or renal dysfunction occasionally caused by ACEI. The combination of the vasodilators **isosorbide dinitrate** (see Chapter 41) and **hydralazine,** although not as effective as an ACEI in prolonging survival, can be used instead of an ACEI or ARB for patients in whom blocking the RAA system is contraindicated. Hydralazine causes mainly arterial vasodilatation, possibly via inhibition of Ca^{2+} release from the sarcoplasmic reticulum.

β-Receptor blockers

The 1993 MDC study reported that the β_1-selective antagonist **metoprolol** reduced mortality when added to conventional therapy for mild to moderate CHF. The benefits of adding metoprolol to standard therapy (ACEI and diuretics) were confirmed in the 1999 MERIT-HF study, which showed that this drug reduced 1-year mortality by 34% in patients with mild to severe CHF. **Bisoprolol,** another β_1-selective antagonist, was shown by the 1999 CIBIS-II trial to similarly diminish mortality. **Carvedilol** is a non-selective β-blocker that has additional α-antagonist and antioxidant properties, and has also been shown to prolong survival in CHF. The 2003 COMET trial showed that when given to patients being treated with ACEI and diuretics, carvedilol extended survival to a greater extent than did metoprolol.

Long-term treatment with β-blockers has been shown to increase ejection fraction, reduce systolic and diastolic volume, and eventually cause regression of left ventricular hypertrophy. Other beneficial effects of β-blockers in CHF probably include reduced ischaemia and a reduction in heart rate, thus improving myocardial perfusion, inhibition of the deleterious effects of excess catecholamines on myocardial structure and metabolism, and reduction of cytokine release. β-Blockers appear to be particularly effective in reducing sudden death in those with CHF, suggesting that the prevention of ventricular fibrillation (see Chapters 48, 50 and 51) constitutes an important part of their action.

The negative inotropic effect of β-blockers is potentially hazardous in some patients with CHF, because cardiac function is already compromised. Therapy is therefore initiated with low doses which are carefully elevated over several weeks or months. Because only the three β-blockers described above have as yet been shown to lengthen survival in CHF, they are the only ones recommended for its treatment.

Ivabradine, although not a β-blocker, also lowers the heart rate (see Chapter 40). The 2010 SHIFT study showed that adding ivabradine to current gold standard treatment significantly reduced death from heart failure in patients with moderate to severe CHF.

Aldosterone antagonists

Aldosterone levels initially fall during ACEI treatment, but often rise again ('escape') during prolonged treatment. Aldosterone has a number of effects that worsen CHF and its consequences: inducing cardiac fibrosis and remodelling, reducing nitric oxide release, increasing Na^+ retention, and promoting arrhythmias by decreasing plasma K^+ and cardiac noradrenaline release.

The aldosterone antagonist **spironolactone** was shown in the 1999 RALES trial to reduce mortality when added to ACEI in severe CHF. Its use is now recommended in patients with more severe heart failure and good renal function. As it can cause hyperkalaemia, careful monitoring of plasma K^+ levels is important.

Spironolactone also causes antiandrogenic side effects such as gynaecomastia. The more selective aldosterone antagonist **eplerenone** is also used, and has fewer side effects.

Diuretics

Diuretics reduce fluid accumulation by increasing renal salt and water excretion. Preload, pulmonary congestion and systemic oedema are thereby relieved. **Loop diuretics** inhibit the Na^+–K^+–$2Cl^-$ symport in the thick ascending loop of Henle. Na^+ and Cl^- reabsorption is thereby inhibited, and the retention of these ions in the tubule promotes fluid loss in the urine. Diuretics are commonly used in CHF, including **furosemide**, **bumetanide**, **torasemide** and **ethacrynic acid**. Thiazide and thiazide-related diuretics (see Chapter 38), particularly **metolazone**, are sometimes combined with a loop diuretic.

Both loop and thiazide diuretics can cause hypokalaemia and metabolic alkalosis because the increased Na^+ retained in the tubular fluid is partly exchanged for K^+ and H^+ in the distal nephron. This process is stimulated by aldosterone (see Chapter 29), and diuretic-induced hypokalaemia can be controlled by an ACEI or an aldosterone antagonist. Hypokalaemia can also be treated with K^+ supplements, or the use of **K^+-sparing diuretics** such as **amiloride** or **triamterene**. These inhibit Na^+ reabsorption in the collecting duct. Long-term use of loop diuretics can result in hypovolaemia, reduced plasma Mg^{2+}, Ca^{2+} and Na^+, and hyperuricaemia and hyperglycaemia. This is more common in the elderly, who may require high doses of diuretics to overcome **diuretic resistance**.

Cardiac glycosides

Cardiac glycosides include ouabain, digitoxin and **digoxin**, which is used most widely. Digoxin improves CHF symptoms, but does not prolong life. Cardiac glycosides inhibit the Na^+ pump in cardiac muscle, thereby indirectly inhibiting the Na^+–Ca^{2+} antiport and thus increasing intracellular Ca^{2+} (see Chapter 12). The rise in Ca^{2+} enhances contractility and shortens action potential duration and refractory period in atrial and ventricular cells by stimulating K^+ channels. Digoxin has been shown to increase baroreceptor responsiveness, thereby reducing sympathetic tone.

Digoxin also acts on the nervous system to increase vagal tone. This slows both sinoatrial node activity and atrioventricular node (AVN) conduction, and can be useful in treating atrial arrhythmias (see Chapter 51). It is therefore mainly used in patients with both CHF and atrial fibrillation.

Even a small (two- to threefold) excess of digoxin over the optimal therapeutic concentration can cause arrhythmias. This occurs because an excessive rise in $[Ca^{2+}]_i$ causes oscillations in membrane potential after action potentials. These **delayed afterdepolarizations** can trigger ectopic beats (see Chapter 48), and at higher doses can cause ventricular tachycardia. Inhibition of the Na^+ pump also decreases intracellular K^+, causing depolarization and facilitating arrhythmias. In addition, excess digoxin can increase vagal tone enough to block conduction at the AVN, and can also raise sympathetic tone, again favouring arrhythmias. Digoxin toxicity is enhanced by hypokalaemia (low plasma K^+), because K^+ decreases the affinity of digoxin for the Na^+ pump. Digoxin also causes toxic gastrointestinal effects, including anorexia, nausea and vomiting. Acute toxicity can be treated with intravenous K^+, anti-arrhythmics (e.g. lidocaine) and digoxin-specific antibodies.

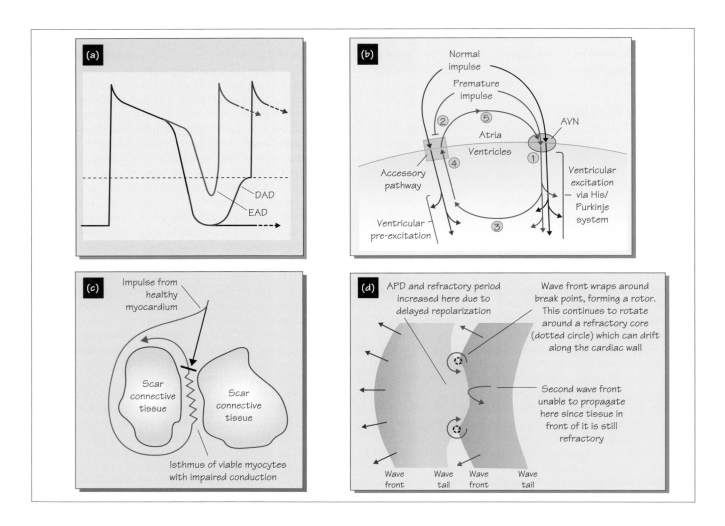

Arrhythmias are abnormalities of the heart rate or rhythm caused by disorders of impulse generation or conduction.

Disorders of impulse generation: latent pacemakers and triggered automaticity

All parts of the cardiac conduction system demonstrate a spontaneous phase 4 depolarization (**automaticity**), and are therefore potential or **latent pacemakers**. Because sinoatrial node (SAN) pacemaking is of the highest frequency (70–80 beats/min), it causes **overdrive suppression** of pacemaking by the atrioventricular node (AVN) (50–60 beats/min) or Purkinje fibres (30–40 beats/min). However, ischaemia, hypokalaemia, fibre stretch or local catecholamine release may increase automaticity in latent pacemakers, which can then 'escape' from SAN dominance to cause arrhythmias.

Triggered automaticity is caused by **afterdepolarizations**. These are oscillations in the membrane potential that occur during or after repolarization. Oscillations large enough to reach threshold initiate premature action potentials and thus heart beats (Figure 48a). This may occur repeatedly, initiating a sustained arrhythmia

either directly or by triggering re-entry (see below). Afterdepolarization magnitude is influenced by changes in heart rate, catecholamines and parasympathetic withdrawal.

Early afterdepolarizations (EADs) occur during the terminal plateau or repolarization phases of the action potential. They develop more readily in Purkinje fibres than in ventricular or atrial myocytes. EADs can be induced by agents that prolong action potential duration and increase the inward current. For example, drugs such as sotalol which block K^+ currents can cause EADs and triggered activity by delaying repolarization, especially when the heart rate is slow. The abnormal rhythms induced by such drugs resemble **torsade de pointes**, a type of congenital arrhythmia.

Delayed afterdepolarizations (DADs) occur after repolarization is complete, and are caused by excessive increases in cellular $[Ca^{2+}]$. DADs can be caused by catecholamines, which increase Ca^{2+} influx through the L-type Ca^{2+} channel, and by digitalis glycosides, which increase $[Ca^{2+}]_i$ (see Chapter 47). They can also occur in heart failure, in which myocyte Ca^{2+} regulation is impaired. The oscillation of membrane potential following the increase in $[Ca^{2+}]_i$ is caused by a **transient inward current** involving Na^+ influx, and the

The Cardiovascular System at a Glance, Fourth Edition. Philip I. Aaronson, Jeremy P.T. Ward, and Michelle J. Connolly.

occurrence and magnitude of DADs and the likelihood that they will cause arrhythmias is increased by conditions that enhance this current. These include increased Ca^{2+} release from the sarcoplasmic reticulum and longer action potentials, which cause larger increases in $[Ca^{2+}]_i$. Therefore, drugs prolonging action potential duration may trigger DADs, whereas drugs shortening the action potential have the opposite effect. The magnitude of the transient inward current is also influenced by the resting membrane potential, and is maximal when this is approximately $-60\,mV$.

Abnormal impulse conduction: re-entry

Re-entry occurs when an impulse that is delayed in one region of the myocardium re-excites adjacent areas of the myocardium more than once. The initiating impulse is often premature, for example having resulted from triggered automaticity. One type of re-entry, termed **anatomical**, requires the presence of three conditions:

1 There must exist an anatomical circuit around which the impulse can circulate (a process termed **circus movement**). This circuit can utilize parallel conduction pathways such as two Purkinje fibre branches, or the AVN and an accessory atrioventricular conduction pathway.

2 Impulse conduction at some point in the circuit should be slow enough to allow the region in front of the impulse to recover from refractoriness. This region is termed the **excitable gap**.

3 The circuit must also include a zone of unidirectional block where conduction is blocked in one direction while remaining possible in the other.

Wolff–Parkinson–White (WPW) syndrome is an uncommon supraventricular arrhythmia (population incidence 0.1–0.2%) which provides a prototypical example of anatomical re-entry (see Chapter 49). People with WPW have a congenital accessory (extra) conduction pathway (formerly termed the **bundle of Kent**) between an atrium and ventricle, which is often situated on the left free wall of the heart. Thus, as shown in Figure 48b, normal atrial depolarization (black arrows) is conducted to the ventricles through both the AVN and the accessory pathway (blue arrows). The accessory pathway has properties differing from that of the AVN. First, it *conducts more rapidly* than the AVN, so the part of the ventricle to which the pathway connects depolarizes before the rest (**pre-excitation**), resulting in a widened QRS complex. Secondly, the accessory pathway has a *longer refractory period* than the AVN. Thus, if a premature impulse arises in an atrium (red arrows), it may be conducted normally to the ventricles via the AVN (**1** in Figure 48), but may not be conducted forwards through the accessory pathway, which is still refractory from the previous impulse (**2**). However, when the impulse through the AVN is distributed to the ventricles (**3**), it will encounter the distal end of the accessory pathway (**4**) which has now had time to recover its excitability, and will be conducted backwards through this pathway into the atrium (**5**). It can then traverse the AVN again and continue to cycle though the anatomical circuit encompassing the AVN, His–Purkinje system, ventricles, accessory pathway and atrium (**1**–**3**–**4**–**5**). The ventricles are excited with each circuit, which causes a tachycardia because the impulse cycles more quickly than the SAN spontaneously depolarizes.

It is noteworthy that the 'border zone' between healthy myocardium and the scar resulting from the healing of a myocardial infarct (see Chapter 44) typically contains a mixture of living muscle cells and connective tissue. In some cases, a narrow band ('isthmus') of still-viable muscle cells spans an area of non-conducting scar, thereby connecting two regions of healthy myocardium (Figure 48c). Conduction of the impulse by the isthmus may be slowed or even demonstrate effective unidirectional block because this tissue takes so long to recover its excitability between action potentials. This arrangement provides conditions analogous to those that WPW (think of the isthmus as playing the part of the accessory pathway and the healthy myocardium to the side of the non-conducting scar as mimicking the AVN), and is thought to cause many ventricular arrhythmias arising in patients following myocardial infarct healing.

Functional re-entry does not require an anatomically defined circuit, and tends to arise when conduction is impaired or repolarization is delayed in a region of myocardium, usually as result of ongoing ischaemia or damage from a previous myocardial infarction. Under these conditions, the firing of frequent or premature impulses can cause the front of one wave of depolarization to collide with the tail of the preceeding wave where it has been slowed (Figure 48d). The second wave is unable to proceed into the region of the myocardium that is still refractory, but at the edges of this region it curls into itself, forming twin 'whirlpools' of depolarization, termed **rotors**. Rotors can similarly form under some conditions if an impulse collides with a structural obstacle such as a scar. Once formed, rotors may persist and continue to emit spiral waves of depolarization with a frequency determined by the rotation period of the spiral; these excite the heart and cause tachycardia. The formation of such spiral waves, and the further fragmentation of the waves of depolarization they generate, is thought to underlie the genesis of the chaotic electrical activity that results in the total loss of atrial or ventricular coordinated contraction termed **fibrillation** (see Chapters 49 and 50).

The sympathetic nervous system and arrhythmias

Sympathetic stimulation of the heart results in results in a variety of β-receptor mediated effects enabling positive chronotropy and inotropy (see Chapters 12 and 13). These include the acceleration of impulse generation and conduction by the SA and AV nodes, respectively. In cardiac muscle cells Ca^{2+} influx and release are facilitated leading to an increased rise in $[Ca^{2+}]_i$ during the action potential, and the activities of multiple ion channels are modulated in such a way as to enhance conduction and decrease refractoriness. These effects are crucial for the normal tuning of cardiac function, but excessive sympathetic stimulation of the heart during myocardial infarction, or in the context of cardiac scarring, ischemia, chronic heart failure or cardiomyopathy, can be arrhythmogenic. The reasons for this are not well understood, but may relate to observations that the myocardium is innervated more densely in some areas than in others and that ion channel expression also varies between different parts of the ventricles. Thus, sympathetic activation may exaggerate intrinsic regional inhomogeneities in conduction velocity and refractoriness. These effects are likely to promote triggered automaticity and functional re-entry and therefore tachycardia and fibrillation.

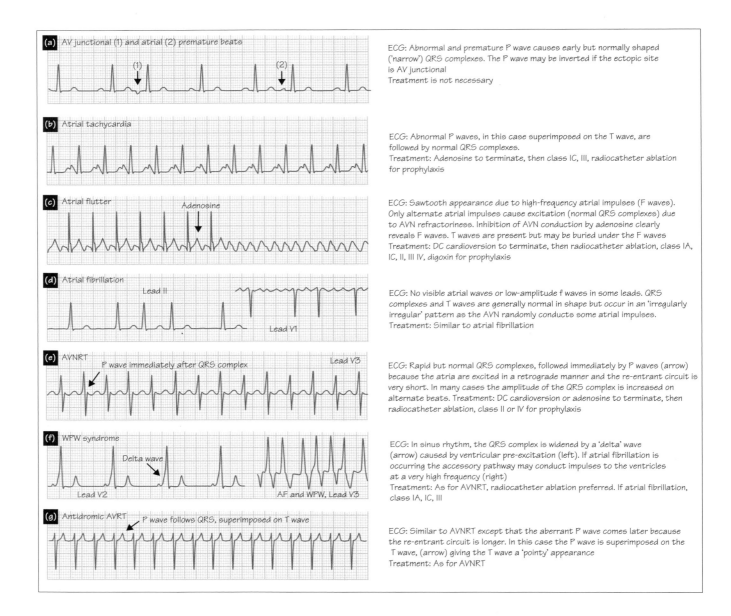

(a) AV junctional (1) and atrial (2) premature beats

ECG: Abnormal and premature P wave causes early but normally shaped ('narrow') QRS complexes. The P wave may be inverted if the ectopic site is AV junctional
Treatment is not necessary

(b) Atrial tachycardia

ECG: Abnormal P waves, in this case superimposed on the T wave, are followed by normal QRS complexes.
Treatment: Adenosine to terminate, then class IC, III, radiocatheter ablation for prophylaxis

(c) Atrial flutter — Adenosine

ECG: Sawtooth appearance due to high-frequency atrial impulses (F waves). Only alternate atrial impulses cause excitation (normal QRS complexes) due to AVN refractoriness. Inhibition of AVN conduction by adenosine clearly reveals F waves. T waves are present but may be buried under the F waves
Treatment: DC cardioversion to terminate, then radiocatheter ablation, class IA, IC, II, III IV, digoxin for prophylaxis

(d) Atrial fibrillation — Lead II / Lead V1

ECG: No visible atrial waves or low-amplitude f waves in some leads. QRS complexes and T waves are generally normal in shape but occur in an 'irregularly irregular' pattern as the AVN randomly conducts some atrial impulses.
Treatment: Similar to atrial fibrillation

(e) AVNRT — P wave immediately after QRS complex — Lead V3

ECG: Rapid but normal QRS complexes, followed immediately by P waves (arrow) because the atria are excited in a retrograde manner and the re-entrant circuit is very short. In many cases the amplitude of the QRS complex is increased on alternate beats. Treatment: DC cardioversion or adenosine to terminate, then radiocatheter ablation, class II or IV for prophylaxis

(f) WPW syndrome — Delta wave — Lead V2 — AF and WPW, Lead V3

ECG: In sinus rhythm, the QRS complex is widened by a 'delta' wave (arrow) caused by ventricular pre-excitation (left). If atrial fibrillation is occurring the accessory pathway may conduct impulses to the ventricles at a very high frequency (right)
Treatment: As for AVNRT, radiocatheter ablation preferred. If atrial fibrillation, class IA, IC, III

(g) Antidromic AVRT — P wave follows QRS, superimposed on T wave

ECG: Similar to AVNRT except that the aberrant P wave comes later because the re-entrant circuit is longer. In this case the P wave is superimposed on the T wave, (arrow) giving the T wave a 'pointy' appearance
Treatment: As for AVNRT

Tachyarrhythmias (tachycardias) and **bradyarrhythmias** (bradycardias) are abnormalities in the origin, timing or sequence of cardiac depolarization that result in a heart rate of >100 and <60 beats/min, respectively. The former are much more common and may be **supraventricular**, in which case they arise in either the atria or the atrioventricular node (AVN), or are **ventricular** in origin (see Chapter 50). Important bradyarrhythmias are described in Chapter 12. Where appropriate, ECG leads that best illustrate the abnormalities associated with each arrhythmia are shown here and in Chapter 50.

Most **supraventricular tachycardias (SVTs)** are troublesome rather than life-threatening, although rarely sudden death can occur. Common symptoms include lightheadedness, palpitations and shortness of breath.

Supraventricular premature beats (Figure 49a) are caused by **ectopic** (i.e. originating from a site other than the SAN) impulses arising in the atria or AVN earlier in the cardiac cycle than would be expected from the normal heart rate. They are typically conducted to the ventricles to cause a premature beat, which is generally followed by a pause as the normal rhythm is reasserted. With an atrial ectopic site the P wave is abnormally shaped because it is not generated in the SAN, and it may be inverted or missing entirely if the ectopic site is in or near the AVN.

The Cardiovascular System at a Glance, Fourth Edition. Philip I. Aaronson, Jeremy P.T. Ward, and Michelle J. Connolly.

Atrial tachycardia heart rate (120–240 beats/min) is frequently caused by an ectopic pacemaker, and can arise in either atrium (e.g. often close to the pulmonary veins in the left atrium). Other atrial tachycardias are re-entrant in nature, frequently following surgery that involves incision into the atrium. The tachycardia may start and stop suddenly or gradually. As with atrial ectopics, the P wave is abnormally shaped (Figure 49b).

Atrial flutter results from re-entry in an atrium (usually the right), often with an area of slowed conduction near the orifice of the inferior vena cava and a circuit involving the whole atrium. The atrial rate is typically ~300 beats/min. As shown in Figure 49c, the AVN is often able to conduct only every other atrial impulse (2:1 AV block) to the ventricles because it is still refractory from the previous impulse, so that the ventricular rate is typically ~150 beats/min. Less commonly, 3:1 or 4:1 block can occur, leading to correspondingly slower rates of ventricular contraction. The ECG has a 'sawtooth' appearance due to the presence of rapid regular **F waves** representing atrial depolarization; these become more obvious if AVN conduction and the QRS complex are suppressed, for example, by adenosine (Figure 49c, right). Atrial flutter is typically seen in patients with underlying cardiac disease, often associated with atrial dilatation. It is particularly common in older hypertensive patients, and may also be caused by acute pulmonary thromboembolism or thyrotoxicosis, but can also develop paroxysmally in patients without underlying heart disease (e.g. secondary to infection or alcohol excess). Attempts to **cardiovert** (restore normal sinus rhythm) atrial flutter with class IA drugs (see Chapter 51) may cause severe ventricular tachycardia and sudden death by establishing 1:1 AVN conduction. This occurs because these drugs suppress vagal firing, thereby increasing AVN conduction. This hazard is avoided by pre-administering a drug that suppresses AVN conduction (e.g. a β-blocker).

Atrial fibrillation (AF) is a chaotic atrial rhythm resulting in an atrial rate of 350–600 beats/min and a lack of effective atrial contraction. The ventricular rate is described as 'irregularly irregular' and is fast but typically less than 200 beats/min because the AVN is unable to conduct most of the atrial impulses impinging upon it (Figure 49d). AF is the most common arrhythmia, occurring in ~10% of people over the age of 75, and has many causes including but not limited to cardiac disease. Initially, AF is often paroxysmal (episodic), but then becomes more persistent, and finally permanent. Paroxysmal AF is usually driven by an ectopic focus or re-entrant pathway in the cardiac muscle layer surrounding pulmonary veins where they enter the left atrium. As AF progresses, it causes changes in the electrical and structural properties of the atrial myocardium, promoting further and more complex forms of re-entry, this rendering the arrhythmia more persistent and refractory to treatment. Palpitations, dyspnoea, dizziness, chest pain or **syncope** (sudden fainting) may occur as a result of the increased ventricular rate or the absence of atrial systolic filling, which reduces ventricular stroke volume by ~20%. Thrombi may form in the left atrial cavity or appendage because the lack of coordinated atrial contraction leads to stasis of blood. These can then embolize to the systemic circulation, particularly the brain and limbs. For this reason, AF is the most important cause of stroke in the elderly.

Pharmacological treatment aims to restore normal sinus rhythm ('rhythm control'); amiodarone is often used for this purpose. A class IV or other agent can also be used to suppress AV conduc-tion, thereby reducing the frequency of impulses that reach and excite the ventricles ('rate control') even if the atria continue to fibrillate.

Atrioventricular nodal re-entrant tachycardia (AVNRT) and **atrioventricular re-entrant tachycardia (AVRT)** result in periodic episodes during which the heart rate abruptly increases to 150–250 beats/min, and they are therefore referred to as **paroxysmal supraventricular tachycardias**. Individuals with AVNRT have an additional or accessory conduction pathway between the atrium and the AVN. In most cases, the normal AV pathway (termed α) conducts rapidly and has a long refractory period, while the accessory (β) pathway conducts slowly and has a short refractory period. In these individuals, AVNRT can be initiated by a premature impulse arising in an atrium. This impulse will not be conducted by the α pathway if it is still refractory from the preceding impulse. However, the impulse may travel slowly down the β pathway (which has recovered from the preceding impulse), and then encounter the distal end of the α pathway. Sufficient time has now elapsed for this pathway to be no longer refractory, and the impulse is able to ascend the α pathway in a *retrograde* (backwards) direction, allowing it to return to the atrium. From here it can continue to cycle through the α and β pathways, exciting the ventricles to cause a heart beat with each circuit. An abnormal P wave is also generated each time the impulse cycles through the atrium. This immediately follows the QRS complex because the re-entrant circuit, and thus the cycle time, is very short (Figure 49e).

An accessory pathway allowing impulse conduction between an atrium and ventricle also exists in AVRT, but in this case it is not located within the AVN. Those in whom this pathway can conduct impulses in both directions may develop **Wolff–Parkinson–White (WPW)** or **pre-excitation syndrome,** the mechanism of which is described in Chapter 48. When the individual is in normal sinus rhythm, the atrial impulse is conducted in an *anterograde* (forward) direction through both the accessory pathway and the AVN. Because it is conducted more quickly through the accessory pathway, excitation of part of one ventricle occurs more quickly than normal (i.e. pre-excitation occurs), resulting in a shortened PR interval and an initial widening of the QRS complex referred to as a *delta wave* (Figure 49f, left). During the tachycardia, however, the accessory pathway conducts in the *retrograde* direction (see Chapter 48) and so pre-excitation does not occur. Instead, premature P waves (often superimposed on the T wave) caused by rapid excitation of the atria by the retrograde impulse are observed. This type of accessory pathway is particularly dangerous in people with atrial fibrillation, because it is often better at conducting rapid impulses than the AVN bevause of its shorter refractory period. Thus, the AVN 'filter' which protects the ventricles from high-frequency atrial activity is bypassed, and the ventricular rate becomes very fast. In this case, the ECG shows rapid and irregular QRS complexes, the majority of which are widened by pre-excitation (Figure 49f, right).

Less common forms of AVRT also exist. In *antidromic* AVRT, the accessory pathway conducts in an anterograde direction during the tachycardia (Figure 49g). In other cases, the accessory pathway is capable of conducting only in the retrograde direction. Thus, pre-excitation does not occur, and the bypass pathway is said to be *concealed*.

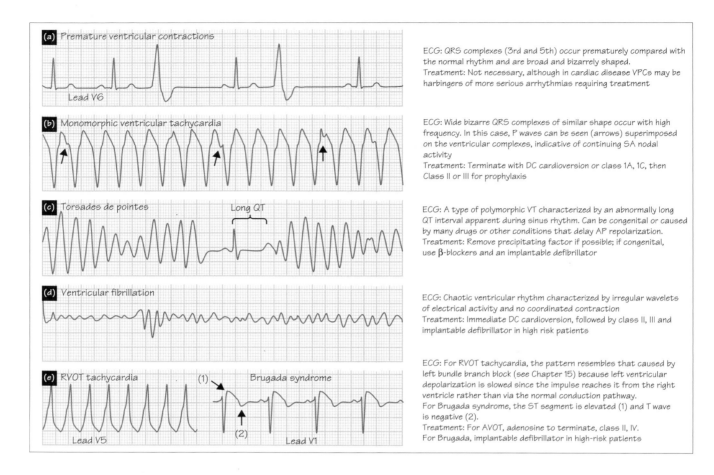

(a) Premature ventricular contractions

Lead V6

ECG: QRS complexes (3rd and 5th) occur prematurely compared with the normal rhythm and are broad and bizarrely shaped.
Treatment: Not necessary, although in cardiac disease VPCs may be harbingers of more serious arrhythmias requiring treatment

(b) Monomorphic ventricular tachycardia

ECG: Wide bizarre QRS complexes of similar shape occur with high frequency. In this case, P waves can be seen (arrows) superimposed on the ventricular complexes, indicative of continuing SA nodal activity
Treatment: Terminate with DC cardioversion or class 1A, 1C, then Class II or III for prophylaxis

(c) Torsades de pointes

Long QT

ECG: A type of polymorphic VT characterized by an abnormally long QT interval apparent during sinus rhythm. Can be congenital or caused by many drugs or other conditions that delay AP repolarization.
Treatment: Remove precipitating factor if possible; if congenital, use β-blockers and an implantable defibrillator

(d) Ventricular fibrillation

ECG: Chaotic ventricular rhythm characterized by irregular wavelets of electrical activity and no coordinated contraction
Treatment: Immediate DC cardioversion, followed by class II, III and implantable defibrillator in high risk patients

(e) RVOT tachycardia

Brugada syndrome

(1)
(2)

Lead V5   Lead V1

ECG: For RVOT tachycardia, the pattern resembles that caused by left bundle branch block (see Chapter 15) because left ventricular depolarization is slowed since the impulse reaches it from the right ventricle rather than via the normal conduction pathway.
For Brugada syndrome, the ST segment is elevated (1) and T wave is negative (2).
Treatment: For AVOT, adenosine to terminate, class II, IV.
For Brugada, implantable defibrillator in high-risk patients

Tachyarrhythmias originating in the ventricles are most often associated with ischaemic heart disease and primary or secondary heart failure (i.e. dilated cardiomyopathies). They are common during and up to 24 h after acute myocardial infarction (MI), when increases in sympathetic activity and extracellular [K⁺] as well as slowed conduction favour their initiation. Such *peri-infarction* arrhythmias may be immediately life-threatening, and indeed the vast majority of deaths associated with MI are caused by ventricular fibrillation occurring before the individual reaches the hospital. If survived, these arrhythmias generally do not recur and are not associated with a subsequent increased risk over and above that conferred by the MI itself. Subsequently, however, the border zone of the healed infarct scar may serve as a substrate for the development of dangerous re-entrant ventricular tachyarrhythmias which can recur or become incessant weeks to years after the MI. Their seriousness and prognostic significance are related to the extent of cardiac damage and impairment of ventricular function that has been sustained. These late arrhythmias themselves confer an additional risk of death, and must be treated either with drugs or with an **implantable defibrillator** (see below). Ventricular tachyarrhythmias can also be associated with cardiomyopathy, and valvular and congenital heart disease, although idiopathic varieties may occur in structurally normal hearts.

Specific ventricular tachyarrhythmias

Premature ventricular contractions (PVCs) are caused by a ventricular ectopic focus and can occur randomly or following every (*bigeminy*; Figure 50a) or every second (*trigeminy*) normal beat. Because depolarization is initiated at a site within ventricular muscle, it spreads throughout the ventricles more slowly than normal impulses which are distributed rapidly by the specialized His–Purkinje conduction system. Thus, the QRS complex is broad and abnormally shaped. PVCs may be of no prognostic consequence, but can predispose to more serious arrhythmias if they develop during or after MI, and/or occur during the T wave of the preceding beat.

Ventricular tachycardia (VT) originates in the ventricles, and is defined as a run of successive ventricular ectopic beats occurring at a rate of >100 beats/min (usually 120–200 beats/min). VT is classified as *non-sustained* or *sustained* based on whether it lasts for >30 s. Depending on the heart rate, VT can cause symptoms such as syncope, angina and shortness of breath, and if sustained can compromise cardiac pumping, leading to heart failure and death. VT can also deteriorate into ventricular fibrillation (see below), particularly with a heart rate of >200 beats/min.

The ECG in VT demonstrates high frequency, bizarrely shaped QRS complexes which are abnormally broadened (>120 ms in duration). Normal atrial activation may continue to be driven by

The Cardiovascular System at a Glance, Fourth Edition. Philip I. Aaronson, Jeremy P.T. Ward, and Michelle J. Connolly.

the SAN (Figure 50b), or the abnormal ventricular pacemaker may cause atrial tachycardia via retrograde impulses traversing the AVN. The configuration of the QRS complex can be used to classify VT into two broad categories. In *monomorphic* VT (Figure 50b), the QRS complexes all have a similar configuration and the heart rate is generally constant, whereas in *polymorphic* VT both the QRS configuration and the heart rate vary continually. Monomorphic VT generally indicates the presence of a stable re-entrant pathway, the substrate for which is typically an MI-related scar (see Chapter 48). Polymorphic VT is thought to be caused by multiple ectopic foci or re-entry in which the circuit pathway is continually varying, and most often occurs during or soon after an MI.

Torsade de pointes ('twisting of the points') is a type of polymorphic VT in which episodes of tachycardia, which may give rise to fibrillation and sudden death, are superimposed upon intervals of bradycardia, during which the QT interval (indicative of the ventricular action potential duration) is prolonged (Figure 50c). During the tachycardia, the ECG has a distinctive appearance in which the amplitude of the QRS complexes alternately waxes and wanes. Torsade de pointes may be caused by drugs or conditions that delay ventricular repolarization (e.g. class IA and III antiarrhythmics, hypokalaemia, hypomagnesaemia). It is also associated with **congenital long QT (LQT) syndrome**, which can be caused by mutations in *KvLQT1* or *HERG*, genes coding for cardiac K^+ channels mediating repolarization, or *SCN5A*, the gene coding for the cardiac Na^+ channel. In congenital LQT syndrome, torsades de pointes is often triggered by sympathetic activity (e.g. caused by stress), which may give rise to early or delayed afterdepolarizations, and may also involve functional re-entry mediated by spiral waves of depolarization (see Chapter 48).

Ventricular fibrillation (VF) is a chaotic ventricular rhythm (Figure 50d) incompatible with a cardiac output which will rapidly cause death unless the patient is resuscitated. VF may follow episodes of VT or acute ischaemia, and frequently occurs during MI. It is the main cause of sudden death, which is responsible for ~10% of all mortality. VF is generally associated with severe underlying heart disease, including ischaemic heart disease and cardiomyopathy.

Focal VT and **fascicular tachycardia** are forms of VT that are idiopathic (i.e. can occur in structurally normal hearts). Focal VT most commonly originates in the **right ventricular outflow tract** (RVOT tachycardia; Figure 50e, left) and is associated with increases in sympathetic activity. This is thought to raise intracellular [cyclic AMP] and therefore $[Ca^{2+}]_i$, initiating delayed afterdepolarizations. Fascicular tachycardia may in some cases be caused by a re-entrant circuit involving the Purkinje system. Idiopathic VTs generally have a good prognosis, and can usually be successfully eliminated with radiofrequency catheter ablation (see below).

VF occasionally occurs idiopathically, for example in people with LQT syndrome or **Brugada syndrome** (Figure 50e, right). This latter condition is associated with ion channel mutations (e.g. in *SCN5A*) which shorten the action potential in epicardial but not endocardial cells of the right ventricle, a situation favouring the development of re-entry.

Non-pharmacological treatment for arrhythmias

Direct current (DC) synchronized cardioversion allows rapid cardioversion (reversion to sinus rhythm) of haemodynamically unstable VT and SVT. Shocks of 50–200 J are delivered in synchrony with the R wave of the QRS complex to the anaesthetized patient via adhesive defibrillator pads placed below the right clavicle and over the apex of the heart.

Radiofrequency catheter ablation (RCA) has assumed a central role in treating many types of arrhythmias. In RCA, the pathways or focally automatic sites causing certain tachyarrhythmias are ablated (destroyed) by focal heating delivered via a catheter. The catheter is inserted through a vein and the tip is located at the surface of the endocardium at the site of the abnormality. Radiofrequency energy is delivered to the tip and dissipated to a large indifferent plate, usually over the back. The tip temperature is set to 60–65°C, resulting in a lesion 8–10 mm in diameter and of a similar depth. This technique is curative in >90% of certain supraventricular arrhythmias. RCA is also increasingly being used to treat VT when an appropriate target site (e.g. a slowly-conducting 'isthmus' in a myocardial scar) can be identified.

Although seldom causing complications, RCA of sites very close to the AV node can potentially cause inadvertent AV nodal damage and therefore permanent block, requiring pacemaker implantation. This can be avoided using **cryoablation,** in which the catheter tip is cooled rather than heated. Cooling the tip briefly to −30°C causes a focal block of electrical activity that is reversible and so cannot cause permanent damage. If this stops the arrhythmia without causing undesirable effects the tip is then further cooled to −60°C, which causes a permanent lesion and ablation of the abnormal rhythm.

Implantable defibrillators consist of a generator connected to electrodes placed transvenously in the heart and superior vena cava. A sensing circuit detects arrhythmias, which are classified as tachycardia or fibrillation on the basis of rate. The treatment algorithm is either as burst pacing, which can terminate VT with a high degree of success, or by the delivery of a shock at up to 40 J, which can cardiovert VT and VF. Shock delivery is between an electrode in the right ventricle and another in the superior vena cava or to the body of the generator (active can). Refinements in detection allow the distinction of supraventricular and ventricular arrhythmias, so that several tiers of progressively more aggressive therapy can be set up. The AVID study reported in 1997 that in patients with malignant ventricular arrhythmia, this approach improved survival by 31% over 3 years compared with antiarrhythmic drug therapy (mainly amiodarone).

Electronic pacemakers can be used either temporarily or permanently to initiate the heart beat by imposing repeated cardiac depolarizations. Temporary pacing is generally accomplished using a catheter-tipped electrode introduced transvenously and provides for the rapid treatment of bradycardias. A temporary pacemaker can also be used to terminate a persistent arrhythmia by pacing the heart at a rate somewhat faster than that of the arrhythmia; sinus rhythm is often restored when this **overdrive pacing** is stopped. Permanent pacemakers are usually implanted to treat bradycardias, for example due to AV block or sick sinus syndrome (see Chapter 13). The pacemaker is implanted under the skin on the chest, and stimulates the heart through leads introduced into the heart transvenously, usually through the subclavian vein. Contemporary pacemakers are able to pace both the atria and ventricles to maintain AV synchronization, and to adjust the pacemaking frequency to respond to changes in physical activity by sensing parameters such as respiration and the interval between the stimulated depolarization and the T wave, a measure of sympathetic nervous system activity.

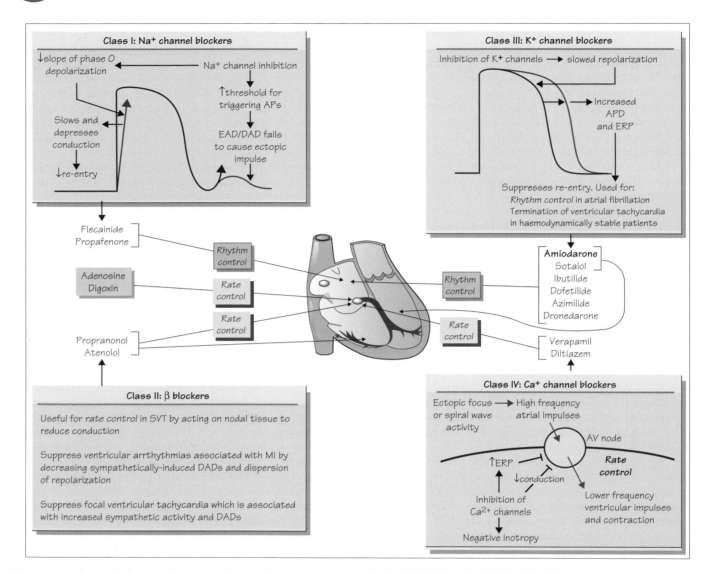

Most anti-arrhythmic drugs, whatever their specific mechanisms, have two actions that reduce abnormal electrical activity, but cause tolerably small effects on normal myocardium.

1 They suppress abnormal (ectopic) pacemakers more than they do the sinoatrial node.

2 They increase the ratio of the effective refractory period to action potential duration (ERP:APD).

Anti-arrhythmic drugs are divided into four classes, based on their mechanisms (Figure 51). However, most anti-arrhythmic drugs have properties of more than one class, often because drug metabolites have their own separate anti-arrhythmic effects or because the drugs exist as 50/50 mixtures of two stereoisomers with different actions. This classification system, introduced by Vaughan Williams and Singh, also excludes several drugs, and is not useful for matching specific drugs to particular arrhythmias. A more clinically relevant classification scheme is shown in Table 51.1.

Clinical trials have shown that class I agents do not enhance survival, and in fact are deleterious if used for some purposes (e.g.

Table 51.1 Site-based classification of anti-arrhythmic drugs.

Atria (*rate control* of SVT)	Classes IC, III
Ventricles	Classes IA, IB, II
AV node (*rhythm control* of SVT)	Adenosine, digoxin, classes II, IV
Atria and ventricles, AV accessory pathways	Amiodarone, sotalol, classes IA, IC

prevention of ventricular ectopic beats). Conversely, the class III agent amiodarone modestly increases survival, and class II agents (β-blockers) can suppress a wide spectrum of arrhythmias and increase survival in conditions such as chronic heart failure and ischaemic heart disease which frequently lead to lethal arrhythmias. However, because radiofrequency catheter ablation can effectively cure many superventricular tachyarrhythmias and implantable defibrillators are more effective than drugs in reducing

The Cardiovascular System at a Glance, Fourth Edition. Philip I. Aaronson, Jeremy P.T. Ward, and Michelle J. Connolly.

the incidence of lethal ventricular arrhythmias, the emphasis of arrhythmia management is shifting towards device-based therapy.

Class I drugs

Class I drugs act mainly by blocking Na^+ channels, thus slowing and depressing impulse conduction. This suppresses re-entrant circuits which depend on an area of impaired conduction, as further Na^+ channel blockade here may block conduction completely, which terminates the arrhythmia. Class I drugs can also suppress automaticity by raising the membrane potential threshold required for delayed afterpolarizations to trigger action potentials (APs).

Because they have a higher affinity for Na^+ channels when they are open or inactivated, these drugs bind to Na^+ channels during each AP and then progressively dissociate following repolarization. Dissociation is slowed in cells in which the resting potential is decreased, and this deepens channel blockade in tissue that is depolarized due to ischaemia.

Three subclasses of class I drugs are designated based their differential effects on the AP in canine Purkinje fibres. Once bound, each subclass of drug dissociates from the Na^+ channel at different rates. Class IB drugs (**lidocaine**, **mexiletine**) dissociate from the channel very rapidly and almost completely between APs. They therefore have little effect in normal myocardium because the steady-state level of drug bound to the channel is minimal. However, in tissue that is depolarized or firing at a high frequency, dissociation between impulses is decreased, promoting channel blockade and depression of conduction. These drugs have therefore been used to treating ventricular tachycardia (VT) associated with MI, which mainly originates in myocardium depolarized by ischaemia. Conversely, class IC drugs (**flecainide**, **propafenone**) dissociate very slowly, remaining bound to channels between APs even at low frequencies of stimulation. This strongly depresses conduction in both normal and depolarized myocardium, thus reducing cardiac contractility. The intermediate dissociation rate of class IA drugs (**procainamide**, **disopyramide**) causes a lengthening of the ERP, which gives them class III activity (see below).

Class I drugs cause many side effects, not the least of which are several types of arrhythmia. This **pro-arrhythmic** effect is unsurprising, given that depression of conduction and prolongation of the AP can induce arrhythmia development (Chapter 48).

At present, class 1B lidocaine and procainamide are sometimes used to terminate episodes of VT. Class 1C drugs (e.g. flecainide, propafenone) are used mainly in the prophylaxis of certain supraventricular tachycardias, particularly AF, and act by suppressing the arrhythmia at its source. This approach to treating SVT is termed **rhythm control**. An alternative approach, **rate control**, uses drugs that slow or block the conduction of impulses through the AVN, thereby slowing the ventricles and unmasking the underlying atrial rhythm. Drugs used for this purpose include class II and IV agents, as well as adenosine and digoxin.

Class II drugs

β-Blockers such as **propranolol** and **atenolol** form the second class of anti-arrhythmics (Figure 51, lower right). They are used for rate control in SVT, and work by reducing the conduction of the atrial impulse through the AVN, because this is promoted by sympathetic stimulation. They can also be useful in ameliorating VT because sympathetic drive to the heart is arrhythmogenic, particularly if there is ischemia or structural heart disease (Chapter 48).

Class III drugs

Class III drugs are K^+ channel blockers that increase APD and therefore prolong ERP. Re-entry occurs when an impulse is locally delayed, and then re-enters and re-excites adjacent myocardium (see Chapter 48). Drugs that prolong ERP can prevent this re-excitation because the adjacent myocardium is still refractory (inexcitable) at the time when the delayed impulse reaches it.

The class III agent amiodarone is effective against both SVT and VT, probably because it also has class IA, II and IV actions. Although amiodarone modestly reduces mortality after MI and in congestive heart failure, its long-term use is recommended only if other anti-arrhythmic drugs fail, because it has many cumulative adverse effects and must be discontinued in about one-third of patients. Hazards include pulmonary fibrosis, hypo- and hyperthyroidism, liver dysfunction, photosensitivity and peripheral neuropathy. Amiodarone also has a very unpredictable and long (4–15 weeks) plasma half-life, which complicates its oral administration. **Dronedarone** is a new class III drug, used to prevent recurrence of AF, which is structurally similar to amiodarone and also has class I and IV activity. Compared with amiodarone, it has fewer side effects and a much better pharmacokinetic profile ($t_{1/2}$ of 1 day) but is less effective. It cannot be used in patients with severe heart failure, and may in rare cases cause liver failure. **Sotalol** is a mixed class II and III drug used for both VT and SVT. Although it causes far fewer extra-cardiac side effects than amiodarone, it is more likely to cause torsades de pointes (see Chapter 50). **Dofetilide**, **ibutilide** and **azimilide** are drugs that are seen as 'pure' class III agents in that they are relatively selective for the voltage-gated K^+ channels involved in repolarization. These drugs are used to terminate atrial flutter and fibrillation. Ibutilide is used to premedicate patients due for cardioversion because it enhances myocardial sensitivity. These agents can also cause torsades de pointes, although azimilide is less apt to do so. **Vernakalant** is a new class III drug used to terminate episodes of AF. It acts selectively on the atria, and seems to cause torsades de pointes less often than other class III drugs.

Class IV drugs, adenosine and digoxin

Class IV drugs (**verapamil**, **diltiazem**) are used to treat SVT, and exert their anti-arrhythmic effects on the AVN by blocking L-type Ca^{2+} channels, which mediate the AVN action potential. Their blockade therefore slows AVN depolarization and conduction, and also increases its refractory period. These effects suppress AVN re-entrant rhythms and can slow the ventricular rate in atrial flutter and fibrillation by preventing a proportion of atrial impulses from being conducted through the AVN. Negative inotropy can occur due to L-type channel inhibition, especially if left ventricular function is impaired. Negative inotropic and chronotropic effects are exacerbated by coadministration of β-blockers. These drugs are also sometimes effective in treating focal ventricular tachycardias, because these may be triggered by DADs (see Chapters 48 and 50).

Adenosine, an endogenous nucleoside (see Chapter 23), acts on A_1-receptors in the AVN, suppressing the Ca^{2+} current and enhancing K^+ currents. This depresses AVN conduction enough to break the circuit causing the tachyarrhythmia. Adenosine, given as a bolus injection, is the drug of choice for rapidly terminating SVT. It commonly causes transient facial flushing, bronchospasm and a sense of impending doom. **Digoxin** slows AV conduction by stimulating the vagus and is used to treat AF and other SVTs, especially in patients with heart failure (see Chapter 47).

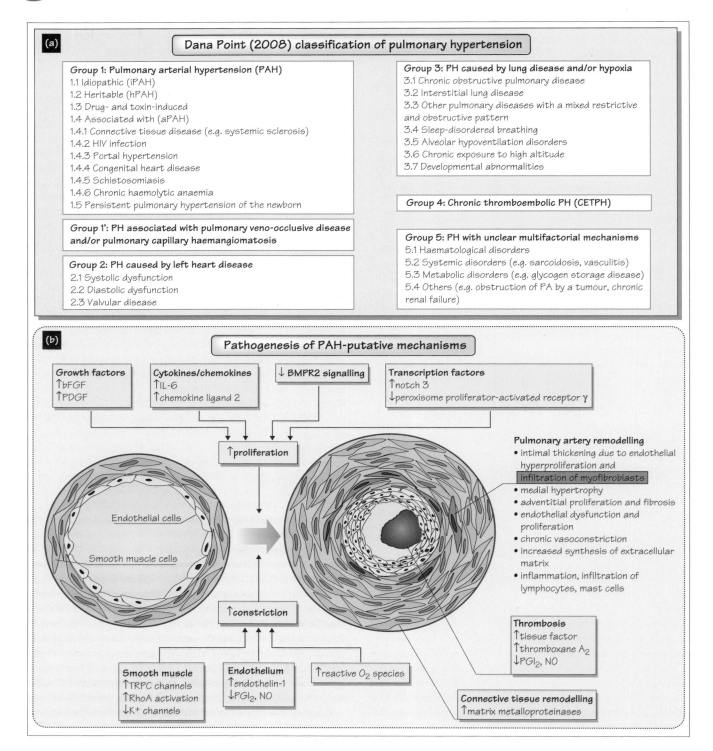

(a) Dana Point (2008) classification of pulmonary hypertension

Group 1: Pulmonary arterial hypertension (PAH)
1.1 Idiopathic (iPAH)
1.2 Heritable (hPAH)
1.3 Drug- and toxin-induced
1.4 Associated with (aPAH)
1.4.1 Connective tissue disease (e.g. systemic sclerosis)
1.4.2 HIV infection
1.4.3 Portal hypertension
1.4.4 Congenital heart disease
1.4.5 Schistosomiasis
1.4.6 Chronic haemolytic anaemia
1.5 Persistent pulmonary hypertension of the newborn

Group 1': PH associated with pulmonary veno-occlusive disease and/or pulmonary capillary haemangiomatosis

Group 2: PH caused by left heart disease
2.1 Systolic dysfunction
2.2 Diastolic dysfunction
2.3 Valvular disease

Group 3: PH caused by lung disease and/or hypoxia
3.1 Chronic obstructive pulmonary disease
3.2 Interstitial lung disease
3.3 Other pulmonary diseases with a mixed restrictive and obstructive pattern
3.4 Sleep-disordered breathing
3.5 Alveolar hypoventilation disorders
3.6 Chronic exposure to high altitude
3.7 Developmental abnormalities

Group 4: Chronic thromboembolic PH (CETPH)

Group 5: PH with unclear multifactorial mechanisms
5.1 Haematological disorders
5.2 Systemic disorders (e.g. sarcoidosis, vasculitis)
5.3 Metabolic disorders (e.g. glycogen storage disease)
5.4 Others (e.g. obstruction of PA by a tumour, chronic renal failure)

(b) Pathogenesis of PAH-putative mechanisms

Growth factors
↑bFGF
↑PDGF

Cytokines/chemokines
↑IL-6
↑chemokine ligand 2

↓ BMPR2 signalling

Transcription factors
↑notch 3
↓peroxisome proliferator-activated receptor γ

↑proliferation

Endothelial cells

Smooth muscle cells

Pulmonary artery remodelling
• intimal thickening due to endothelial hyperproliferation and infiltration of myofibroblasts
• medial hypertrophy
• adventitial proliferation and fibrosis
• endothelial dysfunction and proliferation
• chronic vasoconstriction
• increased synthesis of extracellular matrix
• inflammation, infiltration of lymphocytes, mast cells

↑constriction

Smooth muscle
↑TRPC channels
↑RhoA activation
↓K⁺ channels

Endothelium
↑endothelin-1
↓PGI$_2$, NO

↑reactive O$_2$ species

Thrombosis
↑tissue factor
↑thromboxane A$_2$
↓PGI$_2$, NO

Connective tissue remodelling
↑matrix metalloproteinases

The mean pressure in the pulmonary artery (mPAP) in a normal resting adult is ~16 mmHg. Pulmonary hypertension (PH) is defined as a mPAP exceeding 25 mmHg at rest. The increased PAP can be due to a rise in pulmonary vascular resistance (PVR), increased pulmonary blood flow due to a systemic to pulmonary shunt (Eisenmenger's syndrome; see Chapter 55) or back pressure from the left heart. PH increases right ventricular afterload, eventually leading to right heart failure.

Types of pulmonary hypertension

PH was initially (in 1973) classified as **primary** if it was idiopathic (without a known cause) and **secondary** if a cause could be identi-

The Cardiovascular System at a Glance, Fourth Edition. Philip I. Aaronson, Jeremy P.T. Ward, and Michelle J. Connolly.

fied. More complex classification schemes designed to group the various manifestations of PH according to their pathological and/ or clinical features and management options were then created in 1998, 2003, and most recently at the 4th World Symposium on PH held in Dana Point in 2008 (Figure 52.1, top). Together, the various forms of PH affect ~100 million people worldwide.

Group 1 PH, also termed **pulmonary arterial hypertension** (PAH) comprises heritable (hPAH) and idiopathic PAH (iPAH) and also PH associated with a number of other conditions (aPAH). Patients demonstrate a clinical syndrome indicative of severe PH and an increased PVR associated with a unique set of pulmonary vascular abnormalities (see below). Both hPAH and iPAH are characterized by a decreased expression of **bone morphogenetic protein receptor type 2** (BMPR2) which, usually in hPAH and sometimes in iPAH, is associated with mutations in *BMPR2*, its cognate gene. **Group 1′ PH,** associated with pulmonary veno-occlusive disease and pulmonary capillary haemangiomatosis, has features resembling those of PAH separate clinical entity.

Groups 2–5 are forms of secondary PH. **Group 2 PH** is due to left heart disease, chiefly ventricular failure or mitral and/or aortic valve disease, which results in increased left atrial pressure that backs up into the pulmonary artery. **Group 3 PH** is associated with lung diseases such as chronic obstructive pulmonary disease (COPD) and cystic fibrosis and other conditions such as sleep apnoea, the common factor being the presence of alveolar hypoxia. **Group 4 PH** is associated with chronic thromboembolic disease, with a persistent blockage of pulmonary arteries arising from venous thromboembolism. **Group 5** represents PH associated with a heterogeneous set of conditions such as chronic myeloid leukaemia, sarcoidosis, Gaucher's disease, and thyroid disease. Secondary PH is generally managed by treating the cause. Group 2 PH is often controlled as a consequence of addressing the underlying left heart disease, whereas Group 3 PH patients with COPD may benefit from O_2 therapy. Group 4 PH is treated with anticoagulation and surgical removal of the embolus (thromboembolectomy).

Pulmonary arterial hypertension

PAH includes hPAH and iPAH, as well as severe PH which for unknown reasons often arises in association with certain conditions (aPAH). iPAH and hPAH together affect only ~15 people per million, whereas aPAH is much more common. PAH prognosis is poor, with a 15% mortality rate after 1 year; the only cure is lung transplant. Right ventricular function is an important determinant of prognosis, as patients usually die from progressive right heart failure, and individuals vary with regard to the ability of the right ventricle to compensate for the increased afterload generated as a result of the increased PVR.

Pathophysiology

Although excessive pulmonary vasoconstriction is an important factor in ~20% of PAH cases, the main cause of the increased PVR in PAH is **pulmonary remodelling** characterized by excessive pulmonary artery (PA) smooth muscle cell proliferation. PA remodelling typically results in hyperplasia of the intimal layer due to the invasion of myofibroblasts (cells with properties of fibroblasts and smooth muscle), as well as hypertrophy of the medial layer, and adventitial proliferation. These processes cause the muscularization of very small PA, which normally contain little smooth muscle. Thrombosis *in situ*, inflammation, and the presence of

complex vascular lesions (often termed **plexiform lesions**) comprising endothelial cells, lymphocytes and mast cells, are additional features that contribute to raised PVR and blood flow restriction. The causes of remodelling remain controversial, but some of the mechanisms currently thought to contribute to this process are shown in Figure 52b.

Clinical findings and diagnosis

Often the first clinical manifestation of pulmonary hypertension is gradually increasing breathlessness upon exertion and fatigue. As the condition progresses, these symptoms may be present at rest. Other symptoms include chest pain and peripheral oedema.

Physical examination Signs in severe PH include an increased intensity of the pulmonary component of the second heart sound due to the elevated pulmonary pressure that increases the force of closure of the pulmonary valve and a midsystolic ejection murmur indicating turbulent pulmonary outflow.

Diagnosis PH is best diagnosed via right heart catheterization. A Swan–Ganz catheter is inserted via the femoral vein and advanced into the vena cava and then into the right atrium, right ventricle and finally the pulmonary artery, where the mPAP is measured.

Management

Management of PAH includes treatment of symptoms, and newer specific therapies designed to slow disease progression, but which do not afford a cure. Symptomatic therapy includes diuretics to reduce peripheral oedema, anticoagulants to prevent clots, inhaled O_2 to increase blood oxygenation and digoxin to provide positive inotropy. Calcium-channel blockers can lower PAP in a small subset of patients. Specific therapies include **prostacyclin (PGI_2) analogues**, **endothelin receptor antagonists** and **phosphodiesterase-5 inhibitors**.

Production by PA of PGI_2, an endothelium-derived vasodilator and inhibitor of platelet aggregation, is thought to be deficient in PAH, and stable PGI_2 analogues have become a mainstay of its treatment. **Epoprostenol**, the first to be introduced, is used for the intravenous treatment of advanced PAH, and is the only drug that has been shown to lengthen survival in PAH. **Iloprost** is a synthetic analogue of PGI_2 which is delivered by inhalation.

Endothelin-1 (see Chapter 24) is a potent vasoconstrictor and pro-proliferative agent that may contribute to the development of PAH, inhibition of endothelin receptors has shown promise in its treatment. **Bosentan** is an antagonist of ET_A and ET_B receptors which was shown in the BREATHE-1 trial to significantly improve exercise tolerance. **Ambrisentan**, a selective blocker of the ET_A receptor is also used, and was shown in the ARIES-1 and ARIES-2 trials to improve the 6-minute walk distance (a test often used to gauge the severity of PAH) after 12 weeks.

Production by PA of the potent endothelium-derived vasodilator nitric oxide (NO), which acts by increasing smooth muscle cell cyclic guanosine monophosphate (cGMP) levels (see Chapters 15 and 24), is thought to be deficient in PAH. cGMP is broken down by various phosphodiesterases (PDEs), so that PDE inhibition enhances and prolongs the vasodilating effect of NO. PDE-5 is the most important phosphodiesterase in the pulmonary circulation, and PDE-5 inhibitors (**sildenafil, vardenafil**) have accordingly emerged as an important pillar of therapy. The SUPER-1 study showed that patients taking sildenafil were more likely to show an improvement in symptoms than those taking placebo.

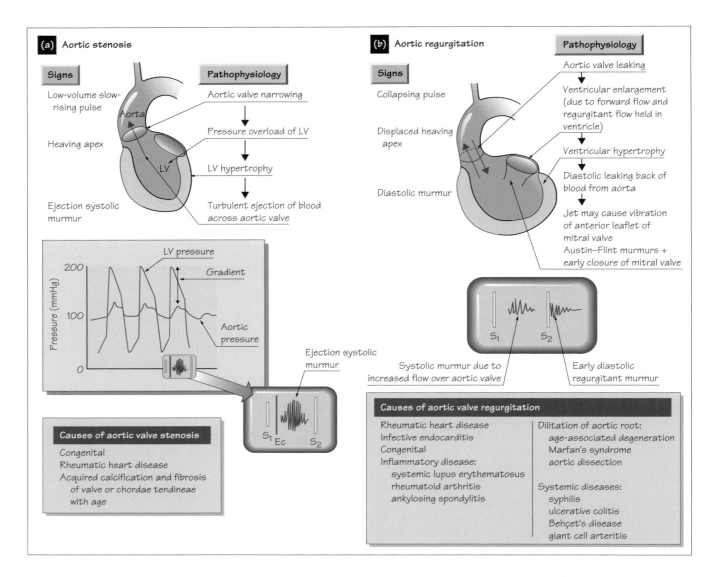

The **aortic valve** links the left ventricle (LV) and the aorta. It is normally tricuspid. Impaired aortic valve opening, due to its narrowing, is known as **aortic stenosis** (AS). It impedes outflow of blood from the LV into the aorta and imposes a **pressure load** on the LV. Deficient valve closure (**aortic regurgitation**, AR, *incompetence*) allows blood to flow back into the LV and thus imposes a **volume load** on the LV.

Aortic stenosis
Causes
Senile calcification This is the most common cause. Calcium deposits occur at the base of the cusp, without involvement of the commissures. This is most likely related to prolonged mechanical stress, and is more common in people with congenital bicuspid valves. About 50% of patients aged under 70 with significant AS have bicuspid valves, whereas most older patients with AS have tricuspid valves.

Rheumatic AS as a result of rheumatic heart disease is unusual without coexisting mitral valve disease. Male sex, diabetes and hypercholesterolaemia are also risk factors for AS.

Congenital A **unicuspid aortic valve** is usually fatal within 1 year of birth. **Bicuspid** aortic valves develop progressive fusion of the commissures, and symptoms usually present after 40 years. Infants with atherosclerosis due to lipid disorders may develop AS in conjunction with **coronary artery disease** (CAD).

Pathophysiology
A slow reduction in aortic valve area requires the LV to pump harder to expel blood into the aorta, which causes **left ventricular hypertrophy** and eventual myocardial dysfunction, arrhythmias and **heart failure** (see Chapter 46). 'Critical' AS occurs when there is greater than a 75% reduction of valve area, to <0.5 cm²/m² body surface area, and a >50 mmHg gradient between peak systolic LV

The Cardiovascular System at a Glance, Fourth Edition. Philip I. Aaronson, Jeremy P.T. Ward, and Michelle J. Connolly.

and aortic pressure at a normal cardiac output. With worsening AS, cardiac output cannot increase adequately during exercise and eventually becomes insufficient at rest. As AS progresses the left ventricle dilates, and LV end-diastolic pressure (EDP) increases to the point where overt LV failure ensues.

Clinical features

AS is typically associated with a triad of symptoms: angina, syncope and breathlessness. Patients present usually between the ages of 50 and 70 years, most commonly with **angina** either due to reduced cardiac output secondary to AS reducing coronary artery perfusion relative to myocardial demand or concurrent CAD (50% have concurrent CAD). In AS the hypertrophied LV has an elevated oxygen demand and inadequate cardiac output for this demand occurs during exercise. Exercise tolerance is decreased, and if cerebral blood flow is insufficient patients may develop **exercise-associated syncope**. Once patients with AS develop angina, syncope or LV failure, their median survival is less than 3 years.

Patients with mild AS have a normal blood pressure and pulse. In moderate to severe AS the pulse is slow-rising and has a narrow pulse pressure. There may be a demonstrable **thrill** (vibration) felt on palpation over the precordium. The apex beat is **heaving** due to LV hypertrophy. Initially, the apex is non-displaced; however, once the LV starts dilating in late-stage AS then it will displace. Auscultation reveals a normal S_1, **a quiet S_2** and an **ejection systolic murmur** (Figure 53a; see Chapter 32), heard best in the second intercostal space on the right and which classically radiates to the carotids. It is louder with squatting and softer with standing or during the **Valsalva manoeuvre** (forced expiration against a closed glottis). With worsening AS and a fall in cardiac output, the murmur may become softer (**silent AS**).

Investigations

The ECG shows LV hypertrophy with strain (ST depression, T-wave inversion). Atrial fibrillation and ventricular arrhythmias are often seen when LV function has deteriorated. Echocardiography shows reduced valve opening and calcification of cusps, and permits calculation of valve area. Doppler imaging allows calculation of the pressure gradient between the LV and aorta.

Management

Many patients with AS are old and have comorbidities – in some cases their symptoms can be conservatively managed as the risks of valve intervention outweigh the benefits. When valve intervention is planned it is important that it is done before the LV starts to dilate. Risk factors for CAD, such as hypertension, and angina symptoms can be treated medically. However, it is important that systemic hypotension and arterial vasodilatation are avoided, so β-blockers and other negative inotropes should be stopped. Cardiac catheterization with **coronary angiography** must be performed prior to valve replacement, and coronary artery bypass performed if significant CAD is present. Several types of mechanical valve are available, including those of a 'ball and cage' variety or tilting disc. These will always require **anticoagulant therapy** (see Chapter 8). Valves can also be obtained from pigs or human cadavers and these have the advantage that anticoagulants are not generally required, hence these can be used in women of childbearing age, because warfarin is teratogenic. **Balloon valvuloplasty** can be performed in children with non-calcified valves, but is of little value in adults.

Aortic regurgitation

AR occurs when the valve cannot close firmly at the end of ventricular systole and as a result blood flows back into the ventricle from the aorta at the start of diastole.

Causes

Causes of AR include **rheumatic disease**, where fibrous retraction of the valve cusps prevents apposition, **infective endocarditis** causing valve damage and **congenital malformations** (e.g. bicuspid valve) (Figure 53b).

Pathophysiology

AR imposes a volume load on the LV because of flow back into the ventricle. **Acute AR** (trauma, infective endocarditis, aortic dissection) is usually catastrophic. Here the LV cannot accommodate the acute increase in volume and LV EDP rises. The early increase in LV EDP causes premature closure of the mitral valve and inadequate forward LV filling, resulting in cardiovascular collapse and acute respiratory failure.

In **chronic AR**, volume load and LV EDP increase gradually, and **LV hypertrophy** allows adequate output to be maintained. As the aortic valve never completely closes, there is no LV isovolumetric relaxation phase (see Chapter 16) and the pulse pressure is wide.

Clinical features

Patients usually do not present with symptoms until LV failure develops. Signs include a wide pulse pressure (caused by reduction in diastolic pressure) and a **collapsing pulse** (see Chapter 16). The LV apex is displaced laterally and is hyperdynamic. Auscultation reveals a high-pitched **early diastolic murmur** at the left sternal edge, and often a **systolic flow murmur** across the aortic valve. AR is associated with several eponymous signs. While these are rare in clinical practice, they are favoured by some finals examiners. **Quincke's sign** is visible nail bed pulsation; **Corrigan's sign** denotes visible pulsations in the carotids; **de Musset's sign** is pulsatile head bobbing; **Traube's sign** is a 'pistol shot' heard on auscultation of the femoral arteries; the **Austin Flint murmur** is a **rumbling late diastolic murmur** caused by premature closure of the mitral valve; it denotes **severe AR**.

Investigations

Echocardiography can determine the aetiology and severity of AR by imaging the valve leaflets and LV dimensions, aortic root diameter and diastolic closure or fluttering of the mitral valve. Doppler imaging quantifies the amount of regurgitation.

Management

Acute severe AR requires urgent valve replacement. Chronic AR has a generally good prognosis until symptoms develop. Patients with moderate AR should undergo echocardiography every 6–12 months. Valve replacement should be considered in symptomatic patients, or in asymptomatic patients with worsening LV dimensions, LV function or aortic root diameter. Valve replacement is similar to that for AS, except that replacement of the aortic root may also be required in patients with a severely dilated ascending aorta.

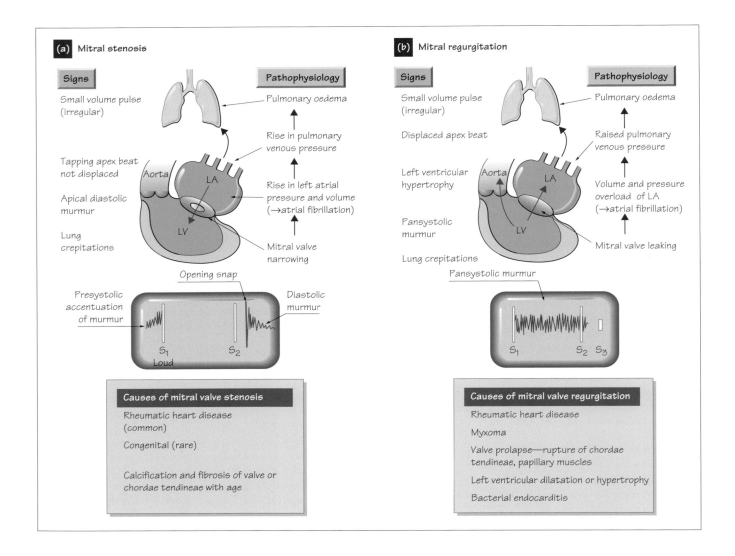

(a) Mitral stenosis

Signs
- Small volume pulse (irregular)
- Tapping apex beat not displaced
- Apical diastolic murmur
- Lung crepitations

Pathophysiology
- Pulmonary oedema
- Rise in pulmonary venous pressure
- Rise in left atrial pressure and volume (→atrial fibrillation)
- Mitral valve narrowing

Aorta, LA, LV

Presystolic accentuation of murmur — Opening snap — Diastolic murmur

S_1 Loud S_2

Causes of mitral valve stenosis
- Rheumatic heart disease (common)
- Congenital (rare)
- Calcification and fibrosis of valve or chordae tendineae with age

(b) Mitral regurgitation

Signs
- Small volume pulse (irregular)
- Displaced apex beat
- Left ventricular hypertrophy
- Pansystolic murmur
- Lung crepitations

Pathophysiology
- Pulmonary oedema
- Raised pulmonary venous pressure
- Volume and pressure overload of LA (→atrial fibrillation)
- Mitral valve leaking

Aorta, LA, LV

Pansystolic murmur

S_1 S_2 S_3

Causes of mitral valve regurgitation
- Rheumatic heart disease
- Myxoma
- Valve prolapse—rupture of chordae tendineae, papillary muscles
- Left ventricular dilatation or hypertrophy
- Bacterial endocarditis

The **mitral valve** is normally bicuspid and separates the left atrium (LA) and left ventricle (LV). The valve may narrow (**mitral stenosis**) or leak (**mitral regurgitation**).

Mitral stenosis
Causes
Mitral stenosis (MS) is usually caused by prior episodes, often during childhood, of acute **rheumatic fever**. This causes thickening and fusion of the mitral **commissures**, **cusps** or **chordae tendineae**, making the cusps less flexible and narrowing the orifice. Symptoms from MS usually develop more than 10 years after the acute attack of rheumatic fever, which patients may not recall. The normal area of a mitral valve is 6cm²; critical MS occurs when this area falls

to 1cm². Other less common causes include congenital mitral stenosis and carcinoid tumours, which are very rare.

Pathophysiology
MS prevents the free flow of blood from the LA to the LV, and slows ventricular filling during diastole. The left atrial pressure rises to maintain cardiac output, and there is **atrial hypertrophy and dilatation**. The elevated left atrial pressure causes pulmonary congestion and can result in **pulmonary hypertension** and **oedema**, and **right heart failure** (see Chapter 46). Patients with MS rely on atrial systole (the so-called 'atrial kick') for ventricular filling, and **atrial fibrillation** (caused by atrial enlargement) significantly reduces cardiac output. The LV is usually normal in MS, but may

The Cardiovascular System at a Glance, Fourth Edition. Philip I. Aaronson, Jeremy P.T. Ward, and Michelle J. Connolly.

be abnormal due to either chronic underfeeding of the LV or rheumatic scarring.

Clinical features

Patients present in their thirties to forties with **dyspnoea**, either on exertion or during situations that raise cardiac output (e.g. fever, anaemia, pregnancy). This is a result of **pulmonary congestion**, which causes the lungs to become stiffer. Patients may present with **palpitations, chest pain, stroke** (via embolization of thrombi) or **haemoptysis** (coughing up of blood). Hoarseness may be present as a result of the enlarged LA compressing the left recurrent laryngeal nerve. Symptoms may be precipitated by atrial fibrillation. The patient's cheeks may appear pinkish – '**malar flush**' or '**mitral facies**', due to slight arterial hypoxia resulting from the reduced cardiac output. The **apex beat** is described as **tapping** and the first heart sound is loud. Auscultation reveals an **opening snap** soon after S_2 that is best heard at the apex, and by a **rumbling mid-diastolic murmur** leading to a loud S_1. The duration of the murmur is related to the severity of the MS. It is brief in mild MS and **pandiastolic** (i.e. lasts for the whole of diastole) in severe MS. When auscultating for the diastolic murmur of MS, ask the patient to lean towards their left side and to hold their breath in expiration. This manoeuvre helps accentuate the murmur as it brings the heart against the thoracic wall and briefly increases left-sided cardiac output. Patients in sinus rhythm may have **presystolic accentuation** of the murmur due to atrial contraction, and a large venous 'a' wave (see Chapter 16). If the mitral valve is completely immobile there may be no opening snap or a loud S_1. As MS becomes more severe, the pulse becomes less prominent, **crackles** are heard on auscultation of the lung bases because of developing pulmonary oedema, and the **jugular venous pressure** becomes elevated.

The ECG may show signs consistent with LA enlargement only, although many patients are in atrial fibrillation. The chest X-ray may show left atrial enlargement with normal left ventricular size, but with increasing severity of MS there may be pulmonary venous congestion, enlarged pulmonary arteries, denoting pulmonary hypertension, and right ventricular enlargement.

Management

Mild MS may require little treatment, although management should include measures to avoid **anaemia** and **tachyarrhythmias** as these may precipitate decompensation and cardiac failure (see Chapter 46). If the patient is in atrial fibrillation, **rate control** with a β-blocker or rate-limiting Ca^{2+} channel blocker is crucial. Anticoagulation must be given to prevent stroke resulting from an embolus arising from the fibrillating atrium. Patients with MS can remain minimally symptomatic for many years, but deteriorate quickly once symptoms worsen. Therefore, **valve replacement** with a mechanical valve, **valvotomy** (surgical separation of commissures) or **balloon valvuloplasty** (the use of a balloon catheter to force cusps open) should be performed in moderately symptomatic patients.

Mitral regurgitation

Causes

Acute mitral regurgitation (MR) is usually a result of **infective endocarditis**, **ruptured chordae tendineae** or ischaemic **papillary muscle rupture**. Chronic MR arises from **myxomatous degeneration** of the mitral leaflets, **mitral valve prolapse** (reversal into atrium) and chronic MR may also develop in any disease causing LV dilatation, so preventing apposition (coming together) of the mitral leaflets, or because of ischaemic dysfunction of the papillary muscles. As MR causes LV dilatation, mitral regurgitation begets further mitral regurgitation.

Pathophysiology

In **acute MR** the LV ejects blood back into the LA, imposing a sudden volume load on the LA during ventricular systole. Left atrial pressure rises suddenly and this is rapidly followed by a rise in pulmonary venous pressure and capillary pressure. This leads to fluid entering the lung interstitium, causing stiffness and dyspnoea, or into the alveoli, causing **pulmonary oedema**.

Chronic MR is characterized by LV dilatation and hypertrophy, and dilatation of the LA. The latter protects the pulmonary circulation from the effects of the regurgitant volume. This form of MR is called *chronic compensated*. However, LA dilatation leads to atrial fibrillation. The fibrillating atrium is liable to develop **thrombi** that may be **embolized** (dislodge and move freely in the blood) causing stroke (see Chapter 8).

MR imposes a diastolic volume load on the LV that causes dilatation, because each systolic stroke volume is composed of a portion that enters the aorta (LV output) and an ineffective portion that re-enters the LA (LV regurgitant volume) and adds to the venous return. The regurgitant volume increases when LV emptying is impaired, such as with aortic stenosis or hypertension.

Clinical features

Patients with mild chronic MR are usually asymptomatic. As MR worsens, patients develop **fatigue, dyspnoea on exertion, orthopnoea** and **pulmonary oedema** as a result of progressive LV failure and elevation of pulmonary capillary pressure (see Chapter 46). The development of atrial fibrillation is common because of dilatation of the LA. Chronic MR is associated with a **pansystolic** murmur, which is heard best at the apex, and which radiates classically to the axilla. S_1 is soft and S_2 is widely split because of an early aortic component. Echocardiography can detect a prolapsing or rheumatic valve, and determine LV size and function. Doppler imaging of the regurgitant jet can assess the severity of MR.

Management

Management is focused on promoting LV emptying into the aorta. Reduction of afterload with **angiotensin-converting enzyme inhibitors** is beneficial (see Chapter 47). Patients with atrial fibrillation receive **anticoagulants** to prevent stroke. A prolapsing valve may sometimes be repaired. Dilatation of the mitral valve ring may be corrected by implantation of an artificial ring. Rheumatic valves and those damaged by endocarditis often need replacement with an artificial valve. Valve replacement is best performed prior to the development of LV dysfunction or pulmonary hypertension, and should always be performed in patients with symptomatic MR despite medical therapy. The risks of surgery are higher in acute MR; however, valve replacement should be performed in patients with uncontrollable heart failure or end-organ failure, even in cases of acute infective endocarditis.

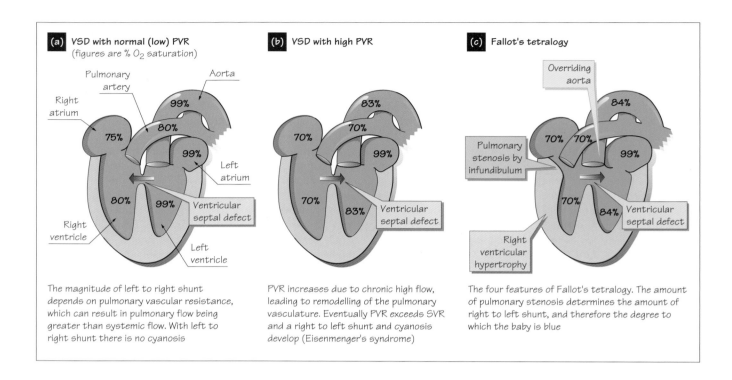

(a) VSD with normal (low) PVR
(figures are % O_2 saturation)

Right atrium
Pulmonary artery
Aorta
99%
80%
75%
99%
Left atrium
80%
99%
Ventricular septal defect
Right ventricle
Left ventricle

The magnitude of left to right shunt depends on pulmonary vascular resistance, which can result in pulmonary flow being greater than systemic flow. With left to right shunt there is no cyanosis

(b) VSD with high PVR
83%
70%
70%
99%
70%
83%
Ventricular septal defect

PVR increases due to chronic high flow, leading to remodelling of the pulmonary vasculature. Eventually PVR exceeds SVR and a right to left shunt and cyanosis develop (Eisenmenger's syndrome)

(c) Fallot's tetralogy
Overriding aorta
84%
Pulmonary stenosis by infundibulum
70% 70%
99%
70%
84%
Ventricular septal defect
Right ventricular hypertrophy

The four features of Fallot's tetralogy. The amount of pulmonary stenosis determines the amount of right to left shunt, and therefore the degree to which the baby is blue

Hypertrophic obstructive cardiomyopathy

Hypertrophic obstructive cardiomyopathy (HOCM) is the most common genetic cardiac disease, with a prevalence of >1 in 500. Although often asymptomatic, it is the leading cause of **sudden cardiac death** in young athletes, and a significant cause in the general population. HOCM is associated with left ventricular hypertrophy, often **asymmetric,** caused by disordered myocardial growth. This is frequently coupled to **dynamic outflow obstruction** as a result of valve dysfunction, conduction defects and arrhythmias. Inheritance is **autosomal dominant.** Mutations in sarcomere-related genes are present in 60% of cases, the most common being β myosin heavy chain (~45%) and cardiac myosin binding protein C (~35%). Clinical features are variable, ranging from asymptomatic through dyspnoea, angina, palpitations and syncope to heart failure, stroke and sudden cardiac death in a minority. Moderate symptoms can be treated with β-blockers and/or verapamil, but in severe cases surgery to relieve the outflow obstruction is required, and high-risk patients benefit from an **implantable cardioverter defibrillator** (ICD).

Channelopathies

Channelopathies are diseases caused by mutations in genes for ion channels, and predispose to arrhythmias, syncope and sudden cardiac death, most commonly in young, otherwise healthy adults with structurally normal hearts.

Long QT (LQT) syndrome is characterized by a prolonged QT interval (QT_C >0.44 s; see Chapter 14). This is normally of no consequence and patients are otherwise healthy, but rarely acute emotion or exertion can trigger the polymorphic ventricular tachyarrhythmia known as **torsade de pointes** (see Chapter 50), causing syncope (most common), seizures or sudden cardiac death. The trigger is increased sympathetic activity (see also CPVT below). LQT syndrome is inherited in an autosomal dominant fashion, with a prevalence of ~1 in 6000; ~4% suffer sudden cardiac death, largely children and young adults, but 30% remain asymptomatic lifelong. In 95% of cases with an identified genetic cause, there are mutations in *KCNQ1* or *HERG*, genes encoding the **delayed rectifier K+ channels** underlying I_K, which is responsible for cardiac action potential repolarization. Most of the rest have mutations in *SCN5A*, encoding the **Na+ channel** (see Chapter 12). Treatment with β-blockers to suppress the effects of sympathetic stimulation is effective, but an ICD may be required. Functional LQT syndrome can be **acquired** in heart failure (see Chapter 46). **Drug-induced** LQT syndrome is common, including class IA and III anti-arrhythmics, but also antimalarial, antihistamine, antibiotic, psychiatric and recreational drugs (e.g. cocaine) because the HERG protein is promiscuous in its interactions. Such drugs dangerously increase risk for genetic LQT syndrome.

Catecholaminergic polymorphic ventricular tachycardia (CPVT) has similar symptoms to LQT syndrome, and is also triggered by acute emotion, exercise and increased sympathetic activity; however, the ECG at rest is normal. Symptoms generally become apparent in the first decade of life, and 60% will have had symptoms by the age of 20. Prevalence may be **1 in 10 000.** Most cases (50–70%) are associated with mutations in *RYR2*, which encodes the **SR Ca²⁺ release channel** and has autosomal dominant inherit-

The Cardiovascular System at a Glance, Fourth Edition. Philip I. Aaronson, Jeremy P.T. Ward, and Michelle J. Connolly.

ance. A minority (~8%) have mutations in *CASQ2*, which encodes **calsequestrin** and is recessive (see Chapter 12). Treatment is the same as for LQT syndrome.

Brugada syndrome is characterized by ST elevation in precordial leads V_1–V_3 (see Chapters 11, 14 and 50). Symptoms usually appear after puberty but can occur at any age, and include syncope, cardiac arrest and sudden cardiac death, often during rest or sleep, as a result of **ventricular fibrillation**. The mean age of sudden death is 40 years. Brugada syndrome is synonymous with *sudden unexplained nocturnal death syndrome*. Inheritance is autosomal dominant, but symptoms are eight- to 10-fold more common in males. Prevalence worldwide may be as high as 1 in 2000, particularly in South East Asia, where it is the leading cause of death in men under 40 apart from accidents. About 30% of cases have been associated with mutations in *SCN5A*, encoding **cardiac Na$^+$ channels**. These lead to shorter action potentials in right ventricle epicardial but not endocardial cells, favouring development of re-entry arrhythmias (see Chapter 50). The only known effective treatment is an ICD.

Congenital heart disease

Congenital heart diseases (**CHDs**) are abnormalities of cardiac structure that are present from birth, caused by abnormal development between 3 and 8 weeks' gestation. The incidence of CHD is ~1% of live births, not including valve disorders such as mitral prolapse or bicuspid aortic valve. Many spontaneously aborted or stillborn fetuses have cardiac malformations, or chromosomal abnormalities associated with structural heart defects. Maternal rubella infection, alcohol abuse and some medications are associated with CHD. CHDs normally present in infancy with either **congestive heart failure** or **central cyanosis**. Congestive heart failure in an infant is usually caused by a **left to right shunt**, such as a **ventricular septal defect** (VSD) or a **patent ductus arteriosus** (PDA), or as a result of aortic obstruction. **Central cyanosis** may be caused by severe pulmonary disease or **right to left shunt**. It is characteristic of **transposition of the great vessels** and **tetralogy of Fallot**.

Ventricular septal defect

VSDs are the most common CHD (0.2% of births), and may occur with other abnormalities. *In utero*, pulmonary vascular resistance (PVR) exceeds systemic vascular resistance (SVR), so most blood exits the left ventricle via the aorta. However, after birth PVR < SVR, and blood is shunted from the left to right ventricle via the VSD, and into the pulmonary artery (Figure 55a). The magnitude of shunt is related to the size of defect and relative size of PVR and SVR. In young children, moderate VSD may limit exercise or cause fatigue, an enlarged heart and hypertrophy. Shunting of blood into the pulmonary circulation leads to pulmonary hypertension, and if persistent irreversible **pulmonary vascular remodelling**. PVR may then exceed SVR, reversing the shunt and causing cyanosis (Figure 55b; **Eisenmenger's syndrome**). Surgical correction is then not possible, so infants with significant VSD benefit from early surgery. Half of smaller VSDs close spontaneously within ~4 years.

Patent (or persistent) ductus arteriosus

PDA may arise because the duct does not close properly due to malformations, possibly related to maternal rubella. It is more common in females. The duct may not close in premature babies due to immaturity. Frequently, PDA is not diagnosed at birth, but only after development of heart failure or infective endocarditis. Treatment is initiated as soon as possible to prevent development of full heart failure. Ligation of the ductus arteriosus must be performed within 5 years of birth. A cyclooxygenase inhibitor to reduce PGE_1 is sometimes sufficient to promote closure.

Transposition of the great arteries

This occurs when the left ventricle empties into the pulmonary artery and the right ventricle into the aorta. It may be associated with VSD, atrial septal defect (ASD) or PDA. The transposition results in two parallel circulations, where deoxygenated systemic venous blood is returned to the body and oxygenated pulmonary venous blood returns to the lungs, causing severe central cyanosis. Unless corrected, it is fatal within 2 weeks for ~30% of cases and within a year for 90%. Surgical correction involves transection of the great vessels and reconnection to their appropriate ventricles. Prior to surgery infants can be stabilized by creation of an artificial ASD, allowing mixing of blood in the atria and oxygenation of systemic blood. Administration of PGE_1 delays closure of the ductus arteriosus and so further access of oxygenated blood to the systemic circulation.

Fallot's tetralogy

The most common cyanotic CHD in children surviving to 1 year (Figure 55c). It consists of a VSD, pulmonary stenosis, an overriding aorta (positioning of aorta over the VSD) and right ventricular hypertrophy. There is a high right ventricular pressure and right to left shunt. The degree of cyanosis depends on the pulmonary stenosis, generally due to misalignment of the infundibulum. Infants with Fallot's tetralogy develop slowly, and may present with dyspnoea, fatigue and hypoxic episodes (**Fallot's or tetralogy spells**), characterized by rapidly worsening cyanosis, progressing to limpness, stroke and loss of consciousness. Surgical correction of the VSD and ventricular obstruction is performed in infancy and has <5% mortality.

Atrial septal defects

ASDs usually go unrecognized until adulthood. They generally involve the midseptum in the ostium secundum and are distinct from a patent foramen ovale. The left to right shunt increases pulmonary blood flow, which if sustained into adulthood leads to pulmonary vascular remodelling and pulmonary hypertension. Adults with ASDs may also have atrial arrhythmias or left ventricular failure. Severe pulmonary hypertension can reverse the left to right shunt and cause right to left shunt and cyanosis. ASDs with significant left to right shunts should be repaired before development of irreversible pulmonary hypertension. Once a right to left shunt has developed, surgical repair is not performed.

Case studies and questions

The following case studies are real examples taken from the author's experience as a junior doctor at a London teaching hospital.

Case 1: A young lady with pleuritic chest pain and shortness of breath

You are the medical house officer on-call and have been asked by the registrar to see a 31-year-old woman, who was referred by her GP complaining of chest pain. Your history-taking reveals that the pain is located in the centre of her chest and that it came on suddenly at rest the day before. It is sharp in character and non-radiating. It is associated with some shortness of breath and a non-productive cough. Deep inspiration exacerbates the pain and it is not relieved by simple analgesia. Upon eliciting her past medical history, you learn that she had recently been in hospital with a fracture of her right femoral shaft. Exploration of her social history reveals that she has smoked 10 cigarettes a day for the past 10 years. Her observations are as follows: temperature 37.2, BP 129/72 mmHg, heart rate 106 regular, respiratory rate 24 and she is saturating at 97% on room air. On examination, she is comfortable at rest and talking in complete sentences. Her hands are warm and well-perfused, and her jugular venous pressure (JVP) is not elevated. Auscultation of her heart reveals normal heart sounds and her chest is clear. An ECG shows sinus tachycardia and her chest X-ray is unremarkable.

1 *Based on the history and your examination, what is the most likely diagnosis?*
2 *What is this patient's pack year history?*
3 *Which investigation would you like to do next?*
4 *Would a D-dimer be a useful investigation in this patient?*
5 *What imaging would you like to do?*
6 *How would you treat this patient?*

Case 2: An elderly woman with a racing heart

You are a foundation year house officer in geriatric medicine. One of your patients, a 98-year-old woman, was admitted from her nursing home with a cough productive of green sputum. She is currently being treated for community-acquired pneumonia with co-amoxiclav and clarithromycin. Three days later, she develops diarrhoea and on the consultant ward round, she complains of a 'racing heart'. The consultant examines her and finds that her mucous membranes are dry and her pulse is 120 irregular. Auscultation of her chest reveals minimal crackles at the left base, and her heart sounds are normal. You ask one of the nurses to record an ECG. You review the ECG and note that the rhythm is irregularly irregular and that P waves are absent. You recall that her admission ECG showed normal sinus rhythm with old ischaemic changes (T wave inversion in V3–V6). You take blood and send it for a full blood count, urea and electrolytes, and C-reactive protein (CRP). You review the bloods and note that the white cell count and CRP are improving but the potassium is 3.0 (normal range 3.5–5.5 mmol/L).

1 *What is the new ECG rhythm?*
2 *What is the likeliest cause of this woman's arrhythmia?*
3 *Why has this woman developed diarrhoea?*
4 *How do you treat this patient?*

Case 3: Diseased heart valve

You are the house officer on the acute medical unit. Overnight an 83-year-old woman has been admitted with chest pain and shortness of breath. On the post-take ward round, the senior house officer on-call that night presents the patient to the consultant. The woman had been feeling unwell and had experienced central chest pain, which was non-radiating. She was short of breath, nauseous, sweaty and clammy. Her past medical history is significant for a coronary artery bypass graft (CABG) in 1989, several non-ST segment elevation myocardial infarctions, atrial fibrillation (AF) and hypertension. Admission bloods were all within normal ranges. Her ECG shows T wave inversion in leads I, aVL and V3–V6 and her chest X-ray shows a raised right hemi-diaphragm and sternotomy wires consistent with her previous CABG. Her blood pressure is 160/90 mmHg. On examination she is comfortable at rest, her pulse is 83 regular, her JVP is not elevated but the character of her carotid pulse is slow-rising. Auscultation of her heart sounds reveals a very quiet second sound and an ejection systolic murmur heard shortly after the first heart sound which is loudest in the second intercostal space in the right upper sternal border and which radiates to both carotids.

1 *What is the most likely diagnosis in this woman?*
2 *Why does she have a soft second heart sound?*
3 *Which investigation would you like to do next?*
4 *How would you treat this woman?*

Case 4: A young man with a new murmur

You are the house officer on a diabetes and endocrine firm. One of your patients is a 34-year-old man, Mr RJ, who was admitted with fever and a rash. On examination, he had a blanching maculopapular rash on the arms, buttocks and lower abdomen, which was itchy. His chest was clear. In view of his fever, you take blood cultures. Four days later the microbiology registrar bleeps you to inform you that the blood cultures have grown Gram-positive cocci. She advises you to start the patient on high dose intravenous flucloxacillin. Each day on the ward round, your SHO examines the patient's chest and notes that it is clear, his heart sounds are normal and that there are no added sounds. The next morning your team agrees to split the ward round and you examine Mr RJ. You note a new early diastolic murmur that is high in pitch. Your own registrar is concerned at this development and requests that you arrange a transthoracic echocardiogram (TEE). The echo reports thickening of the aortic valve and the presence of a moderate to severe jet of aortic regurgitation. Additionally, a small ventricular septal defect was noted. Your registrar then requests that you arrange an urgent transoesophageal echocardiogram (TOE). The TOE revealed that the patient had an aortic root abscess.

1 *What does 'Gram-positive' mean?*
2 *Which organism has most likely been isolated on blood cultures?*
3 *What is your diagnosis?*
4 *How do you further manage Mr RJ?*
5 *What is a ventricular septal defect?*

The Cardiovascular System at a Glance, Fourth Edition. Philip I. Aaronson, Jeremy P.T. Ward, and Michelle J. Connolly.

Case 5: Jugular venous pressure up to the jaw

You are 2 weeks into your new job as a foundation year house officer in geriatric medicine. An 84-year-old woman has been transferred to your hospital for rehabilitation following a successful tissue aortic valve replacement at a tertiary centre. On examination she is comfortable at rest, her hands are cool and her JVP is elevated to her jaw. Corneal arcus is present. Inspection of her precordium reveals a fresh midline sternotomy scar that is healing well. Her apex beat is located in the sixth intercostal space, mid-axillary line. Auscultation of her precordium reveals normal heart sounds. Her chest is notable for stony dullness at the left base and bibasal crepitations. She has pitting oedema to her thighs. ECG shows rate-controlled atrial fibrillation and her chest X-ray shows cardiomegaly, bilateral bat's wing shadowing and bilateral pleural effusions (Case 5 figure). On the ward round, she complains of a poor night's sleep and being 'unable to catch my breath'. A recent echocardiogram showed an ejection fraction of 35%.

1 *What is the JVP a measure of?*
2 *Which vessel are we looking at when we assess the JVP?*
3 *What is corneal arcus?*
4 *Is her apex beat displaced?*
5 *What is the diagnosis in this woman?*
6 *What do cardiomegaly, bibasal shadowing and the pleural effusion on her chest X-ray represent?*
7 *How do you manage this patient?*
8 *Do all patients with cardiac failure have a reduced ejection fraction on echocardiogram?*

Case 6: 'I think he's having a heart attack'

It is the bank holiday weekend and you are the medical house officer on-call. The sister on the coronary care unit bleeps you to see a patient: 'Doctor, can you come right away to see Mr CB. He is a 51-year-old man who is complaining of chest pain. He underwent coronary artery bypass grafting 1 month ago. I think he's having a heart attack.' She reads you his observations, which are

temperature 36.9, BP 146/89 mmHg, pulse 110, oxygen saturations 97% on air, respiratory rate 20.

1 *What do you ask sister to do for the patient immediately?*
   On arrival, you see that the patient is clammy and is wincing in pain with his fist clenched across his chest.
2 *What do you do?*
3 *Do you give this patient a β-blocker?*
4 *Which ECG changes, if present, would you be most concerned about? If these were present, what would you do?*
   Blood test reveals an elevated troponin level.
5 *What is your ongoing treatment plan for this patient?*
6 *What is the next investigation?*
7 *What is the relevance of an elevated troponin level?*

Case 7: A middle-aged smoker with chest tightness

You are the medical house officer on-call. It is a busy take and your registrar asks you to see the next patient, an overweight 58-year-old male office worker who was referred by his GP complaining of chest tightness. You elicit the history of this man's chest tightness and discover that it is located in the centre of his chest and that it is 'squeezing' in nature. It came on as he broke into a sweat while running after his dog the previous day and subsided when he sat down to catch his breath. He tells you it 'went up to my jaw'. Further questioning reveals that he has hypertension and hypercholesterolaemia. He is taking amlodipine (5 mg/day) and simvastatin (20 mg/day). His social history is significant for a 20 pack year history and he drinks 30 units of alcohol per week. His blood pressure is 149/82 mmHg.

1 *What is the most likely diagnosis given the history?*
2 *What risk factors (modifiable and non-modifiable) for coronary artery disease does this man have?*
3 *What is amlodipine?*
4 *What is simvastatin?*
5 *What modifications would you make to this man's existing therapies?*
6 *What long-term treatment should he receive for angina?*

Case 8: A young woman with idiopathic pulmonary arterial hypertension

Dr Gabor Kovacs, Professor Horst Olschewski
Department of Pulmonology, Medical University of Graz, Austria; Ludwig Boltzmann Institute for Lung Vascular Research, Graz, Austria

A 42-year-old woman was referred to our pulmonary hypertension clinic. She sometimes experienced episodes of dyspnoea since the birth of her second child 10 years previously. Although she was physically active, her exercise tolerance had decreased such that she preferred to take the lift to her first floor office.

Physical examination was unremarkable except for a loud second heart sound. According to the patient, this had been discovered a few years ago, but was not investigated further. ECG showed right axis deviation and incomplete right bundle branch block. Chest X-ray showed a dilated pulmonary segment, increased diameter of the central pulmonary arteries, and cardiomegaly (Case 8 Figure). CT of the chest showed a dilated right atrium and right ventricular hypertrophy. Routine lung function testing including CO diffusion capacity revealed normal values. A lung perfusion scan was normal.

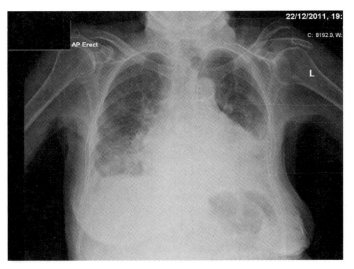

Case 5 AP erect film. Bilateral pleural effusions with adjacent lung atelectasis and generous cardiac silhouette. Sternotomy wires *in situ*. There is also separation of the left acromioclavicular joint.

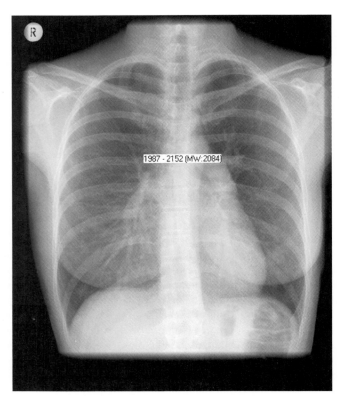

1987 – 2152 (MW:2084)

Case 8 AP erect film. There is increased diameter of the central pulmonary arteries and cardiomegaly.

Echocardiogram showed a normal left atrium and ventricle and no signs of valve disease. The right atrium was dilated and the right ventricular wall was hypertrophic. There was also leftward deviation of the septum. There was minimal tricuspid insufficiency. Given these indirect echocardiographic signs of pulmonary hypertension, the patient underwent right heart catheterization, which revealed severe pulmonary arterial hypertension (PAH) with compensated right ventricular function. Following administration of nitric oxide (NO), the mean pulmonary arterial pressure dropped significantly without a relevant decrease in cardiac output; this was a positive vasodilatator response to NO and thus the patient was deemed an 'NO responder'.

Given the increased pressure in her pulmonary arteries following right heart catheterization and the absence of any cause for her symptoms, a diagnosis of idiopathic pulmonary arterial hypertension (iPAH) was made. As this woman exhibited a positive vasodilator response to NO, therapy with a high-dose calcium-channel blocker (amlodipine) was initiated. Since receiving amlodipine the patient has reported being able to climb the stairs instead of taking the lift. Her cardiomegaly decreased, indicating a decreased pressure load on her right heart.

1 *What is the most frequent presenting complaint of PAH?*
2 *Which is the most important non-invasive investigation in the diagnostic work-up of PAH?*
3 *Which investigation is needed for the definitive diagnosis of PAH?*
4 *Which PAH patients should be treated with high-dose calcium-channel blockers?*

Case studies answers

Case 1 – A young lady with pleuritic chest pain and shortness of breath

1 In a patient with this presentation, you must exclude pulmonary embolism (PE), because this is potentially life-threatening. The nature of this lady's pain – worse on inspiration (i.e. pleuritic) – is typical of PE. The shortness of breath is also in keeping with this diagnosis. This patient has a significant risk factor for a PE: her recent hospitalization (and therefore immobility) with a fracture. Her examination findings (or rather lack thereof) are typical for PE. The most common ECG tracing in PE is sinus tachycardia. In large PEs, signs of right ventricular strain may be present on the ECG. The classic sign of right ventricular strain (and favoured by some finals examiners!) is an S wave in lead I, and a Q wave and T wave inversion in lead III (the so-called $S_1Q_3T_3$ pattern), but this is rare. There may be some right axis deviation and right bundle branch block.

2 Number of pack years = packs smoked per day multiplied by number of years. One pack year = 20 cigarettes/day for 1 year. She has smoked 10 cigarettes/day for 10 years so her pack year history is $0.5 \times 10 = 5$ pack years.

3 An arterial blood gas sample should be taken from the radial artery. This indicates whether or not the patient is hypoxaemic ($pO_2 < 8\,kPa$) or hypocapnic ($pCO_2 < 4.5\,kPa$). In high-risk settings such as postoperative patients, a low pO_2 in combination with dyspnoea, in the absence of other explanations, has a strong positive predictive value for PE.

4 D-dimer is a fibrin degradation product that is released by the body's fibrinolytic system in the process of dissolving the fibrin matrix of a fresh venous thromboembolism. In the investigation of suspected PE, D-dimer has a strong negative predictive value, but a weak positive predictive value. This means in patients with a low clinical probability of PE, a normal D-dimer strongly suggests the absence of a clot but a raised D-dimer warrants further investigation. Other pathologies can also cause a raised D-dimer. However, a raised D-dimer is not helpful in patients in whom PE is the most likely diagnosis from the history and examination, as a normal D-dimer does not exclude a PE in a high-risk patient. Therefore, a D-dimer level would *not* be a useful investigation in this patient.

5 Imaging of the pulmonary vasculature is the gold standard means of diagnosing PE. A CT pulmonary angiogram (CTPA) is performed at the earliest opportunity.

6 Treatment of PE initially consists of anticoagulation with subcutaneous injections of low molecular weight heparin (e.g. tinzaparin or dalteparin). Most hospitalized patients are given venous thromboembolism prophylaxis with reduced dose heparin. If PE is suspected or diagnosed, the patient receives the *treatment* dose of low molecular weight heparin, which is much higher and is calculated according to body weight. After PE is confirmed on CTPA, the patient is started on 6 months' treatment with warfarin to achieve an international normalized ratio (INR) of 2–3.

Case 2 – An elderly woman with a racing heart

1 This patient is now in atrial fibrillation (AF) with a fast ventricular response. Fast because the rate is greater than 100. Atrial fibrillation because the rhythm is irregularly irregular and there are no P waves; recall that the P wave represents organized atrial depolarization and thus contraction.

2 The likeliest causes of this patient's arrhythmia are hypokalaemia and dehydration secondary to diarrhoea.

3 This patient has most likely developed diarrhoea secondary to the antibiotics that she was receiving for her pneumonia.

4 Her serum K^+ and other electrolytes must be corrected. In many cases oral potassium supplements are most appropriate, however, her dry mucous membranes suggest she is dehydrated – a slow bag of intravenous fluids containing 40 mmol/L potassium should be considered in this case. Stopping her antibiotics should be discussed with a microbiologist. Although these reversible factors likely precipitated this episode of AF, her ECG suggests underlying ischaemic heart disease. She may have paroxysmal AF and may not revert to sinus rhythm once her electrolytes are corrected. The long-term management of paroxysmal atrial fibrillation is with anticoagulants (although this is inappropriate if she is at high risk of falls), and either rhythm-control or rate-control agents.
See Chapters 48 and 51.

Case 3 – Diseased heart valve

1 This woman's presentation with this cardiac murmur is most in keeping with aortic stenosis (AS). The classic triad associated with AS is dizziness (presyncope), dyspnoea and chest pain; this woman has two of these. Patients who present with dyspnoea (as opposed to others of the triad) have the poorest prognosis because dyspnoea often indicates an already failing left ventricle. The most common cause of AS is senile calcification of the aortic valve, which generally occurs after the age of 70, although in patients with a congenital bicuspid valve the onset is earlier.

2 This woman's second heart sound is soft because of the poor mobility of the cusps of her aortic valve – her calcified heart valves both open and close poorly.

3 This woman underwent an echocardiogram to assess the degree of stenosis, and corresponding function of her left ventricle. The echo report revealed a heavily calcified, restricted aortic valve with an aortic valve area of $0.4\,cm^2$. A valve area of less than $0.8\,cm^2$ is considered to be severe AS.

4 The only definitive treatment of AS is replacement of the diseased valve. Without valve replacement, survival is less than 3 years. This woman is on the waiting list for a transcatheter aortic valve implantation (TAVI), an alternative treatment to conventional surgical valve replacement. Catheter access to the aortic valve is achieved via the femoral artery or vein, or surgically via a mini-thoracotomy. A replacement valve is inserted through the catheter and placed over the diseased valve, resulting in its obliteration. TAVI is considered in patients who are too high risk for conventional surgery.
See Chapter 53.

Case 4 – A young man with a new murmur

1 Gram-positive means that bacteria have stained dark blue on Gram's staining – they retain the stain owing to the high amount of peptidoglycan in their cell walls. In contrast, Gram-negative organisms have a much thinner peptidoglycan cell wall and therefore do not stain dark blue.

2 The organism that has been isolated on blood cultures is *Staphylococcus aureus*, a Gram-positive coccus which is the primary pathogen of infective endocarditis.

3 This man has infective endocarditis, which is an infection of the endocardial surface of the heart that may include one or more heart valves. *A fever and a new murmur is infective endocarditis until proven otherwise.* Infective endocarditis is extremely serious – the infected heart valves can fail leading to cardiac failure and infected emboli can damage other organs.

4 Mr RJ must continue his course of high dose intravenous antibiotics. In view of his aortic root abscess, Mr RJ required an aortic valve replacement. Repair of his ventricular septal defect was also undertaken.

5 A ventricular septal defect (VSD) is a hole in the septum that separates the ventricles of the heart, resulting in communication between the ventricles with the result that blood flows from the LV to the RV (left-to-right shunt). A significant VSD can be diagnosed clinically by auscultation of a harsh pansystolic murmur at the left sternal border. The consequence of a left-to-right shunt is that, over time, the pressure in the pulmonary circulation increases and pulmonary hypertension develops.
See Chapters 32 and 55.

Case 5 – Jugular venous pressure up to the jaw

1 The JVP is a clinical measure of pressure in the right atrium.

2 The internal jugular vein.

3 Corneal arcus is the name for white rings around the edge of the iris in the eye. They are caused by deposits of cholesterol-rich lipid particles that are thought to be trapped in the extracellular matrix in the stroma of the corneae. Unlike xanthelasmas, they do not indicate an increased risk of ischaemic heart disease or myocardial infarction.

4 This woman's apex beat is displaced. This is a result of cardiomegaly secondary to left ventricular failure. Normally, the apex beat is located in the fifth intercostal space, mid-clavicular line.

5 Her raised JVP and peripheral oedema are signs of right heart failure, while pleural effusions and pulmonary oedema are signs of left heart failure. The diagnosis is therefore congestive cardiac failure.

6 Cardiomegaly occurs as a result of cardiac dilatation in a compensatory attempt of the failing heart to maintain cardiac output. Bilateral bat's wing shadowing represents pulmonary oedema (i.e. fluid in the air spaces) and parenchyma of the lungs causing impaired gas exchange and shortness of breath. The pleural effusions represent excess fluid that has accumulated between the parietal and visceral pleura as a result of increased capillary hydrostatic pressure.

7 This patient was grossly fluid-overloaded. She was started on diuretic therapy to offload the excess fluid, aiming for a weight loss of 0.5–1.0 kg/day. Initially she was started on intravenous frusemide at a dose of 80 mg/day. This was then switched to oral frusemide. She was advised not to drink excessive amounts of fluid. She had daily blood tests to monitor her kidney function, as over-aggressive diuresis can precipitate renal failure. Aggressive diuresis can also cause electrolyte imbalance (e.g. hypokalaemia). If this occurs, the potassium-sparing diuretic spironolactone can be considered. In view of her aortic valve replacement, she should have a repeat echocardiogram to assess the function of her left ventricle.

8 Many patients with cardiac failure have an ejection fraction within normal limits when estimated by echocardiography. This is partly because echocardiogram can only estimate ejection fraction. More importantly, in many patients the heart functions poorly because of problems with filling rather than ejecting out blood into the arterial circulation – this is often called diastolic cardiac failure. *See Chapters 46 and 47.*

Case 6 – 'I think he's having a heart attack'

1 You ask her to sit the patient up and start him on oxygen (initially at 5 L/min) via face mask, perform a 12-lead ECG, put the patient on a cardiac monitor and give two puffs of sublingual glyceryl trinitrate (GTN).

2 You explain you are the on-call doctor and you ask the patient's name. You ask where the pain is – he says in the centre of his chest. He says it feels like someone is 'sitting on my chest'. You ask whether it radiates and he says, 'Yes, down my left arm.' Because prolonged use of high-flow oxygen is no longer recommended in the management of the acute coronary syndromes (ACS), you titrate his oxygen requirements according to his oxygen saturations. You briefly examine him. The ECG shows normal sinus rhythm with T wave inversion in the lateral leads and old pathological Q waves, consistent with a previous myocardial infarction. You ask one of the nurses to administer 5 mg diamorphine with 10 mg metoclopramide (an anti-emetic), give 300 mg aspirin and 300 mg clopidogrel, and then start a GTN infusion. You compare the ECG with the patient's admission ECG and are relieved to note that there are no acute ischaemic changes. Afterwards you document everything in the patient's notes and inform your senior.

3 He has angina, is tachycardic and not in acute cardiac failure. A β-blocker is indicated in this patient, because β-blockers decrease myocardial oxygen demand and therefore limit infarct size. After checking that the patient is not asthmatic, you prescribe a dose of metoprolol.

4 Given this patient's significant cardiac history, you would be most concerned about new ST segment elevation, indicating acute ischaemia that would require urgent revascularization with percutaneous coronary intervention (PCI). If the ECG did show ST segment elevation or depression, you must discuss with your senior and with a cardiologist at a centre that has the capacity for PCI – in a major acute coronary event time is of the essence and he may need emergency transfer to a cardiac centre.

5 This patient has had an ACS. His troponin level measured 6 hours later was elevated having been normal on admission. However, the ECG showed no ST segment elevation. He has therefore suffered an non-ST segment elevation myocardial infarction (NSTEMI). Remember that significant cardiac necrosis can occur without ST segment elevation. He was started on the ACS protocol of drugs: 75 mg/day aspirin and 75 mg/day clopidogrel (both antiplatelet agents) and an antithrombin such as a low molecular weight heparin or 2.5 mg/day fondaparinux. He remained on the cardiac monitor and had repeated ECGs for the duration of his hospital stay.

6 The next investigation in patients with ACS is imaging of the coronary arteries with intervention if necessary. The question is what method of imaging and how soon. This patient's background and positive troponin means he is at high risk of having an unstable coronary artery plaque and therefore needs prompt investigation. He underwent repeat angiography of his coronary arteries.

7 In ACS an elevated troponin level indicates the patient has a high risk of having another coronary event soon and needs urgent further management. However, other pathologies can cause a positive troponin test and not all high risk coronary syndromes have raised troponin levels. An elevated troponin level is *not* diagnostic but should be considered in the context of the patient's history, ECG and other investigations.

See Chapters 42–44.

Case 7 – A middle-aged smoker with chest tightness

1 This man has angina. This is a central chest tightness, or crushing sensation that is due to myocardial ischaemia. The pain of angina may radiate to one or both arms (more commonly the left), to the jaw, neck or back.

2 Modifiable: increased body mass index, sedentary (office worker), hypertension, hypercholesterolaemia, smoking, excessive alcohol intake (28 units/week is the maximum recommended intake for men).

Non-modifiable: male gender.

3 Amlodipine is a long-acting calcium-channel blocker (CCB) belonging to the dihydropyridine class which is used to treat hypertension and angina. It works by relaxing vascular smooth muscle, thus causing a reduction in peripheral vascular resistance, thereby lowering blood pressure. This reduction in peripheral vascular resistance is also thought to explain its efficacy against angina, because this would reduce the afterload against which the heart must pump, thus reducing myocardial oxygen demand.

4 Simvastatin is a statin, a class of lipid-lowering drugs that inhibit HMG-CoA reductase, the enzyme responsible for the rate-limiting step in the synthesis of cholesterol in the liver.

5 His elevated blood pressure reading suggests that his hypertension is not adequately controlled with the low dose of 5 mg/day amlodipine. However, it would be unwise to increase the dose of a long-term antihypertensive based on an isolated BP reading. This man should be given a dose of metoprolol (a β-blocker) and his antihypertensive should be changed to a β-blocker the following day. Simvastatin 20 mg/day is a low dose. In view of his strong risk factors for coronary artery disease, this can comfortably be doubled to 40 mg/day.

6 Most important are lifestyle modifications to reduce his cardiovascular risk factors. He should be encouraged to lose weight, engage in brisk daily exercise and be referred to a smoking cessation clinic. Anti-anginals such as β-blockers, which decrease myocardial oxygen demand, and drugs to halt the progression of his coronary artery disease are essential. He is already taking amlodipine for hypertension and he could continue to take this at an increased dose to treat his angina also. In terms of secondary prevention, he is already taking simvastatin, but the dose of this should be increased. He should be started on 75 mg/day aspirin, which has been shown to decrease mortality. To treat the symptoms of angina, he should be given a GTN spray for sublingual administration prior to any exertion, or to terminate an angina attack. He should be told that if the chest pain is not relieved 5 min after two puffs under the tongue, then he should administer a further two puffs. If this fails to resolve his symptoms, then he should be told to call an ambulance, as he could be suffering an acute coronary event.

See Chapters 40 and 41.

Case 8 – A young woman with idiopathic pulmonary arterial hypertension

1 The most frequent presenting complaint of the disease is shortness of breath on exertion and decreased exercise tolerance. At diagnosis, over 90% of patients report it.

2 The echocardiogram. It allows the estimation of pulmonary arterial pressure and provides information on right ventricular anatomy and function. In our case, a dilated right atrium, a strongly hypertrophic right ventricular wall and leftward septal deviation served as indirect signs of pulmonary hypertension.

3 Right heart catheterization must be performed in order to diagnose PAH.

4 Only those with a positive vasoreactivity test, which is defined as a decrease in mean pulmonary arterial pressure by at least 10 mmHg and to an absolute value that is less than 40 mmHg with unchanged or increased cardiac output following administration of NO.

Concluding remarks

Although idiopathic pulmonary arterial hypertension is generally associated with a very poor clinical outcome, this woman belongs to a small group of patients with an excellent prognosis, provided that the vasodilating calcium-channel blocker is permanently applied at a high dose.

See Chapter 52.

Index